MW00851651

Chinese Medicine Dietetics
Volume 1

To melani: thank you for support my book ! 3-9-12

Prof. Jeffrey C. Pang, L.Ac.
Adam L. White, L.Ac.

www.healthcmi.com
Continuing Education Online
Healthcare Medicine Institute

1st Edition, February 2012

Manufactured in the USA

ISBN-13: 978-0615592428
ISBN-10: 0615592422

Table of Contents

About the Authors

Prof. Jeffrey Pang, L.Ac. received his MD in biomedicine and Traditional Chinese Medicine from Sun Yat Sen University of Medical Science in Guangzhou, China. Since 1984, Prof. Pang has served as the Department Chair for both the theory and herbology departments at Five Branches University. He is a licensed acupuncturist & herbalist and author for the Healthcare Medicine Institute (HealthCMi).

Adam White, L.Ac., Dipl.Ac. (NCCAOM) is a licensed acupuncturist and herbalist, Diplomate of Acupuncture and CEO of HealthCMi. He has served as a faculty member and continuing education director for Five Branches University. His publications cover a variety of topics including Chinese medicine dietetics, the treatment of pelvic inflammatory disorder and herb-drug interactions.

HealthCMi
www.healthcmi.com

The Healthcare Medicine Institute (HealthCMi) provides online continuing education courses to acupuncturists and nurses. HealthCMi is an approved continuing education provider for acupuncturists in the USA, Canada and Australia. HealthCMi courses are pre-approved by the California Acupuncture Board, the NCCAOM (National Certification Commission for Acupuncture and Oriental Medicine), Florida Board of Acupuncture, Texas Medical Board and meets Canadian standards for CTCMA (British Columbia) and CAAA (Alberta) acupuncturist continuing education credit.

Medical professionals download course materials, take an online quiz and receive a certificate of completion online. HealthCMi publishes continuing education online courses in the PDF format to ensure access to course materials on any platform: Apple Macintosh, Windows PC, Linux, iPad and many smart phones including the iPhone and Android cell phones. PDF documents are a secure e-book format that provides medical professionals with the advantage of the search function within continuing education course materials. Clinically, this translates into easy reference to course information for use in the medical setting.

Chinese Medicine Dietetics
Volume 1

History

The Divine Farmer's Herb-Root Classic
Shen Nong Bencao

Although this work was compiled during the Western Han Dynasty, this book's authorship is attributed to Shen Nong who lived approximately 5,000 years ago. Many scholars write that this book was written in the 2nd century CE. It is considered the first major dietetics and herbal medicine book.

Zhou Dynasty (1046-256 BCE) Doctors

1 **Veterinarian**

2 **External injury doctor**
   The Warring States period during the Zhou dynasty required many of these doctors due to combat injuries.

3 **Regular doctor**
   Herbal medicine, acupuncture, and other Chinese medicine

4 **Dietetics doctor**
   These doctors developed a history of working with the chef of the king and are similar to the nutritionists of today. This is a Shi Di (preventative) doctor.

Qin Dynasty (221-206 BCE)

Emperor Qin Shi unified China in 221 BC. Qin Dynasty (221-206 BCE) was the first unified and ruling dynasty of Imperial China and introduced the building of the Great Wall of China. Some scholars attribute the initial writing of the Neijing (Yellow Emperor's Inner Cannon) to the Qin Dynasty. The Neijing is the compilation of two books. The first is the Suwen and the second is the Lingshu. Both works comment on dietetics. Historically, the Suwen (Questions of Organic and Fundamental Nature) makes some of the very first written commentaries on flavors:

1   Excess sour intake causes over-activity of the Liver and hypofunction of the Spleen.

2   Excess saltiness weakens the bones and may cause muscle contracture and atrophy. Excess saltiness causes Heart Qi stagnation.

3   Excess sweet intake causes the Heart Qi congestion and restlessness. Excess sweets imbalances the Kidneys and causes the face to become black.

4   Excess bitter intake disturbs the transforming and transporting function of the Spleen. Excess bitter causes Stomach distention and impairs digestion. Excess bitter intake disturbs the muscles and tendons.

Tang

Tang originally referred to soup and was later used to describe medicinal herb tea. Tang originates from a reference to dietetics soup.

Dietetics Patients

1   Children

Food tastes better than herbal medicinals thereby increasing compliance. Also, children often have weaker Kidney Qi and medicinal teas may be too strong.

2   Elderly

The Kidney Qi is weaker in the elderly and therefore many herbs are too strong. Dietetics provides a gentle alternative.

3   Chronic disease patients

Patients take herbs for a period of time and then may require time off from consuming herbs for clinical reasons. In the interim, it may be advantageous to use dietetics. In addition, patients may desire a break from taking herb tea because they tire of cooking and consuming them. Dietetics provides a way to supply foods with medicinal functions while the patient has a break from the herb tea.

Dietetic Preparations

1   Fresh juice

This treatment is also common in western dietetics. Common use involves fruits and vegetables.

Examples of fresh juice treatments

- Wu Zhi Yin (Five Juice Drink): This drink moistens and tonifies Yin. Regionally, there are several variations on the five ingredients. Conceptually, this drink is fresh vegetable juice often containing herbal ingredients. A basic combination is fresh lotus root, daikon, water chestnut, Asian pear and carrot. Other combinations include fresh Lu Gen juice and fresh Mai Men Dong juice.

Fresh lotus juice, Ou Zhi, is included in some herbal formulas to stop bleeding and tonify Yin. It is available in supermarkets such as Lion Market and Ranch 99.

Li Zhi, Asian pear juice, is especially helpful for children with a dry cough due to climactic dryness in the autumn. During cold weather, the use of home and office heating systems may cause dryness with heat in the air. Breathing dry heat causes dry throat and coughing with blood. Easting Asian pears, Asian pear juice, and other Yin foods are indicated.

Ma Ti (Chinese water chestnut) clears heat, promotes body fluids, and dissolves phlegm. It is sweet, cold, and enters the Stomach, Lung, and Liver channels. It is used in Wu Zhi Yin (Five Juice Drink) for thirst due to heat and body fluid depletion but may also be combined with cucumber and tomato for a similar function.

Freshness is important for the juices. Packaged vegetable and fruit juice products involve more processing and possible additives, which may alter or diminish the function of the juice. In Chinese dietetics, simple is better.

Watercress, Xi Yang Cai, has a strong cooling medicinal function. Watercress shares a similar name to that of American Ginseng (Xi Yang Shen) because of its venerable medicinal properties. Watercress is considered to be a cancer preventative food. A recent study of tobacco smokers notes, "Watercress is a rich source of phenethyl isothiocyanate (PEITC), an effective chemopreventive agent for cancers of the lung and esophagus induced in rodents by nitrosamines, including the tobacco-specific carcinogen 4-(methylnitrosamino)-1-(3-pyridyl)-1-butanone."[1]

2   Yao Cha (Medicinal Tea)

Yao Cha is the mixing of tea leaves with medicinal herbs. In the Chinese medicine clinic, ground and cut herbs are combined with tea (Camellia sinensis) and are added to teabags.

Weight loss teas are popular and include formulations such as the mixing of cha (Camellia sinensis) with Jue Ming Zi,

---

[1] Effects of Watercress Consumption on Urinary Metabolites of Nicotine in Smokers, Stephen S. Hecht2, Steven G. Carmella and Sharon E. Murphy, Cancer Epidemiology, Biomarkers & Prevention October 1999 8; 907.

He Ye, and Shan Zha. There are many pre-made weight loss teabag formulations. However, there are many types of obesity therefore standard teas are not as effective as customized teas based on a differential diagnosis.

Tea has been associated with anticancer properties. One study notes that, "Available epidemiologic evidence supports the hypothesis that increased green tea consumption may be inversely associated with risk of breast cancer recurrence."[2] Another study notes that "our findings provide some support for the hypothesis that tea consumption reduces the risk of ovarian cancer."[3]

3   Kou Fu Ye

Kou means mouth and ye means liquid. Translated, this means taken by oral solution or taken orally. This type of drink is usually a cooked herb that is sterilized and put into a glass ampule. Often, these drinks come with straws. The straws can be inserted directly into the ampule. Ren Shen Kou Fu Ye is popular. This is ginseng that is decocted, sterilized and put into an ampule with liquor. Feng Wan Jiang is another drink, a combination of royal jelly with either Huang Qi or Ren Shen and then put into an ampule with liquor added.

4   Yao Jiu

Yao means herbal medicine and jiu is translated as alcohol. Bai jiu (white alcohol) and Huang Jiu (yellow alcohol) are usually made from rice and are at least 40 proof. This is the strength of brandy and vodka. This strength of alcohol has a

---

[2] Breast Cancer Res Treat. 2010 Jan;119(2):477-84. Epub 2009 May 13. Green tea consumption and breast cancer risk or recurrence: a meta-analysis. Ogunleye AA, Xue F, Michels KB. Department of Epidemiology, Harvard School of Public Health, 677, Huntington Avenue, Boston, MA, USA.

[3] Cancer Causes Control. 2010 Sep;21(9):1485-91. Epub 2010 May 20. Tea consumption and risk of ovarian cancer. Nagle CM, Olsen CM, Bain CJ, Whiteman DC, Green AC, Webb PM. Genetics and Population Health, Queensland Institute of Medical Research, PO Royal Brisbane Hospital, Brisbane, QLD, Australia.

natural ability to kill bacteria thereby allowing for the safe storage of herbs in this form. Herbs are typically soaked in the alcohol for approximately one month for extraction purposes.

This type of formula preparation is mostly used when the functional properties of alcohol are desirable. Alcohol is warming, improves the circulation of blood and 'goes through' the channels (opens the channels).

Common uses include putting an herbal mixture into the alcohol or just ginseng. Many formulas are made by a martial arts shifu (master/teacher) typically for injury recovery and strengthening the body purposes. It is not uncommon to store this type of formula in a large jar. Another formula is made by putting three types of snakes into the alcohol for purposes of opening channel blockages. This is often used for the treatment of arthritis. This formula is known for its dramatic appearance. Since the alcohol is warming, it is common to see this type of preparation used for the treatment of cold and deficient arthritis pain. Wu Jia Pi and Mu Gua are common ingredients.

5   Tang (Soup)

Tang is the major form of dietetic treatment. It is similar to herb tea but something tasty is added. The use of the word tang as soup does not have the decoction meaning as is used for herbal formulas that are outside of the realm of dietetics.

Dang Gui Sheng Jiang Yang Rou Tang: This soup is made by double boiling lean goat meat (Yang Rou, Rou = meat) with Dang Gui, ginger, and Hong Zao (red date). This soup is prized for its flavor and has a very warming temperature. Therefore, it is more appropriate in the winter and not often served in the summer.

6   Yao Zhu and Yao Fan

Zhu is translated as congee and fan is a type of fried rice noodle. Fan is often spelled *fun* as in dishes such as *chow fun* served at Chinese restaurants. Congee, a form of rice soup, is also served at many restaurants but is less common than fan in the USA.

Yao Zhu (congee)
Hui Shan Yao Gou Qi Zi Gu is a healthy congee made with Gou Qi Zi and Shan Yao.

Yao Fan (noodle)
One noodle recipe is made by combining steamed rice, quail, Dang Shen, frog and Shan Yao in a rice cooker combined with rice and water. Once cooked, it is formed into the noodle.

7   Tang Shui (Sugar Soup)

Shui is translated as water. One example of a sugar soup is Lian Zi Bai He Tan Shui. This is made by combining dried lotus seed (which is astringent and tonifies the Spleen) with dried Bai He (which calms the spirit). Soak the herbs and cook until soft. Next, add Bing Tang (rock sugar) to the water. This is often consumed after dinner and helps improve the quality of sleep. Other ingredients commonly added to the Lotus Seed Dried Lily Bulb Soup are Hong Zao (red dates) and white cloud ear fungus (Bai Mu Er).

8   Mi Gao

Mi is honey and gao is a thick syrup, paste, or jelly. Mi Gao is a thick honey syrup with herbs added. Pi Pa Gao is a common cough syrup and typically has pi pa ye (loquat leaf) with herbs such as Yuan Zhi and Xing Ren added to strengthen the stop coughing and dissolve phlegm functions. Another preparation is to boil loquat fruit, add stop coughing herbs, and then add a lot of honey to preserve the dietetics formula. The dual function of honey, to both preserve and add flavor, makes this syrup a valuable component of Chinese medicine dietetics.

Another form of gao is **Gui Ling Gao**. Translated as Turtle Essence Jelly, this medicinal dessert is known for its benefits to the skin and overall complexion. To make Gui Ling Gao, turtle shell is cooked for many hours. Next, herbs such as Tu Fu Ling and ginseng are added to the jelly-like residue. Gui Ling Gao is available in pre-packaged cups, bowls, and pop-top cans and is also available in concentrated powder form. Inexpensive brands of Gui Ling Gao do not contain turtle shell and most brands use farmed turtles and not wild endangered species of turtles.

9   Yao Bing (Cracker, Wafer)

Herbs and medicinal foods can be prepared in a cracker / wafer form. This is popular with children.

Shan Zha (hawthorn berry) is prepared in a wafer form, which is often consumed with herbal medicines to offset bitterness. Shan Zha is sour, treats meat stagnation and this wafer is consumed to benefit digestion. Some brands of hawthorn wafers contain undesirable additives such as food coloring. Gourmet quality hawthorn wafers are occasionally available at Chinese supermarkets.

10   Yao Gao

Yao Gao is a medicinal pastry or cake. Gao refers to pastry or cake in this medicinal preparation. Primary forms of Yao Gao are steamed buns and breads.

Shan Yao Gao is traditionally a steamed bun made from powdered Shan Yao (wild mountain yam, Chinese yam) but it may also be a bread. The dough is made with the powder of Shan Yao, which can be mixed with other powders made from Lian Zi, Shan Zha, various herbs, potatoes and other types of yams. Together they form the starchy flour needed to make Yao Gao.

11   Chai Yao

Chai Gao is the main course of the meal. This is the incorporation of herbs and medicinal foods into cuisine.

One well known dish is Dong Chong Xia Cao (cordyceps) that is double boiled with duck. First, eat the duck and then drink the soup. Dong Chong Xia Cao is valued for its ability to tonify the Lung and Kidney and for stopping coughing with bleeding due to deficiency.

12   Candy

Herbal lozenges for cough, sore throat, and dry throat are some of the most popular herbal candies. Ricola, a Swiss brand of herbal candy, is a popular example in the western world. Bo He and similar herbs are common to herbal candies.

Dietetics and Seasons

Spring

Spring is a time for germination and growing. Things are changing to the color green. The Sheng Bu treatment principle is harmonious with this season. Sheng is translated as raise up and bu is tonify, therefore, raise the Yang Qi upwards. The raising properties of sheng ma make this herb a good choice in the spring. Other herbs such as Dang Shen and Huang Qi are also good choices because they tonify Qi and have a slightly warm temperature. This, too, is harmonious with the Sheng Bu principle of springtime.

Summer

Summer is an ideal time for the Qing Bu method, which clears heat. Use cooling foods when the environment is hot. Eat less fried, dried, and spicy foods. Watercress is an excellent summer choice. For children, it is convenient to clear the heat by cooking Xiao Ku Cao with water. Boiled Xiao Ku Cao has minimal flavor and sugar can be added to make it more appetizing. Ju Hua is another popular choice for clearing heat.

Long Summer

This is an overlapping period at the end of summer and the beginning of autumn. The Dan Bu (Bland Tonify) method is harmonious with long summer. Dan Bu promotes urination to drain dampness and was developed in Southeast Asia where the climate has rains, floods, and even typhoons in the long summer. In the USA, however, climates vary and may not harmonize with the Dan Bu method in long summer. California, for example, has a dry climate at this time of year and the Dan Bu principle is not as relevant as in other regions where heavy rains often occur during long summer.

Dan is translated as bland or as having no flavor. This is represented in the name of the herb Dan Zhu Ye, an herb with little flavor. Fu ling is another example of a bland herb appropriate for the Dan Bu method. Bland herbs usually have a promote urination function which balances long summer's dampness.

Dong Gua Zi (winter melon seed) is used in herbal medicine. In dietetics, the interior white flesh of the winter melon is used. The winter melon is a large, vine grown fruit that has an oval shaped, green exterior similar to that of watermelon. The white of the melon does not have much flavor but it is an excellent choice for both summer and long summer because it clears heat and drains dampness. Often, it is pre-cut when sold in supermarkets. Mild flavors are the key to promoting urination in the long summer. The following dong gua recipe follows the Dan Bu method.

Boil the white, winter melon flesh with Yi Yi Ren. Add herbs such as Chen Pi, Lian Zi, and Qian Shi. Next, add one of the following meats to the soup: chicken, pork, or dried scallops. This soup promotes urination and helps drain the dampness of the rainy season from the body.

Autumn

The Ping Bu (Peaceful Tonify) method gently moistens and tonifies to address dry autumn climactic conditions. Herbs such as Sha Shen, Yu Zhu, and Tai Zi Shen are appropriate. This incorporates the Run Zhao (moisten dryness) method.

Winter

Winter's cold makes the Zi Bu / Wen Bu (Warming Tonify) method appropriate for this season.

Foods such as ginger, cinnamon, goat meat, and deer meat are appropriate choices for winter because they strongly warm to nourish the body. Dang Gui Sheng Jiang Yang Rou Tang is a warming winter dish. This soup is made by double boiling lean goat meat with Dang Gui, ginger, and red dates.

The Five Colors of Food

Five Elements Theory

Red is for the Heart

Most red foods benefit the Heart and the Heart is related to blood. Therefore, red foods generally benefit the Heart and blood. Red is a yang color and therefore many red foods are warming. Examples of healthy red foods include red wine, tomato, and pomegranate.

Western science now finds **red wine** beneficial to the heart. A 1995 study conducted by the University of Toronto, Canada notes that red wine's components trans-resveratrol and quercetin inhibit platelet aggregation. The study notes that the findings "are consistent with the notion that trans-resveratrol may contribute to the presumed protective role of red wine against atherosclerosis and CHD (coronary heart disease)."[4] Another study conducted by

---

[4] Pace-Asciak C.R., Hahn S., Diamandis E.P., Soleas G., Goldberg D.M., "The red wine phenolics trans-resveratrol and quercetin block human platelet aggregation and eicosanoid synthesis: Implications for protection against coronary heart disease," (1995) Clinica Chimica Acta, 235 (2), pp. 207-219.

the University of California, Davis, CA and the Volcani Center, Bet Dagan, Israel, notes that red wine lowers LDL cholesterol:

> The "French paradox" (apparent compatibility of a high fat diet with a low incidence of coronary atherosclerosis) has been attributed to the regular drinking of red wine. However, the alcohol content of wine may not be the sole explanation for this protection. Red wine also contains phenolic compounds, and the antioxidant properties of these may have an important role. In in-vitro studies with phenolic substances in red wine and normal human low-density lipoprotein (LDL) we found that red wine inhibits the coppercatalysed oxidation of LDL. Wine diluted 1000-fold containing 10 μmol/L total phenolics inhibited LDL oxidation significantly more than α-tocopherol. Our findings show that the non-alcoholic components of red wine have potent antioxidant properties toward oxidation of human LDL.[5]

Studies link **tomato** intake with a reduced risk of cardiovascular disease and cancer. A recent study from the School of Public Health, University of North Carolina, Chapel Hill notes:

> Considerable evidence suggests that lycopene, a carotenoid without provitamin A activity found in high concentrations in a small set of plant foods, has significant antioxidant potential in vitro and may play a role in preventing prostate cancer and cardiovascular disease in humans. Tomato products, including ketchup, tomato juice, and pizza sauce, are the richest sources of lycopene in the US diet, accounting for >80% of the total lycopene intake of Americans.[6]

The Department of Nutritional Sciences, Faculty of Medicine, University of Toronto, published:

> At present, the role of lycopene in the prevention of CHD (coronary heart disease) is strongly suggestive. Although the antioxidant property of lycopene may be one of the principal

---

[5] Frankel E.N., Kanner J., German J.B., Parks E., Kinsella J.E., "Inhibition of oxidation of human low-density lipoprotein by phenolic substances in red wine," (1993) Lancet, 341 (8843), pp. 454-457.

[6] L. Arab, S. Steck, "Lycopene and cardiovascular disease1,2,3," Am J Clin Nutr, June 2000 vol. 71 no. 6 1691S-1695S.

mechanisms for its effect, other mechanisms may also be responsible.[7]

The Journal of the National Cancer Institute published that tomatoes are linked to lowering the risk of cancer:

> The epidemiologic literature in the English language regarding intake of tomatoes and tomato-based products and blood lycopene (a compound derived predominantly from tomatoes) level in relation to the risk of various cancers was reviewed. Among 72 studies identified, 57 reported inverse associations between tomato intake or blood lycopene level and the risk of cancer at a defined anatomic site; 35 of these inverse associations were statistically significant. No study indicated that higher tomato consumption or blood lycopene level statistically significantly increased the risk of cancer at any of the investigated sites. About half of the relative risks for comparisons of high with low intakes or levels for tomatoes or lycopene were approximately 0.6 or lower. The evidence for a benefit was strongest for cancers of the prostate, lung, and stomach. Data were also suggestive of a benefit for cancers of the pancreas, colon and rectum, esophagus, oral cavity, breast, and cervix.[8]

Pomegranate has been linked to a decrease in LDL cholesterol, atherosclerotic lesions, and demonstrates anticancer properties. A year 2000 study from the Rambam Medical Center, Haifa, Israel notes:

> In humans, pomegranate juice consumption decreased LDL susceptibility to aggregation and retention and increased the activity of serum paraoxonase (an HDL-associated esterase that can protect against lipid peroxidation) by 20%.... Finally, pomegranate juice supplementation of E^0 mice reduced the size of their atherosclerotic lesions by 44%...."[9]

---

[7] A.V. Rao, "Lycopene, tomatoes, and the prevention of coronary heart disease," Exp Biol Med (Maywood) 2002 November; 227(10): 908–913.

[8] E Giovannucci, "Tomatoes, tomato-based products, lycopene, and cancer: review of the epidemiologic literature," J Natl Cancer Inst. 1999 February 17; 91(4): 317–331.

[9] Aviram M, Dornfeld L, Rosenblat M, Volkova N, Kaplan M, Coleman R, Hayek T, Presser D, Fuhrman B., "Pomegranate juice consumption reduces oxidative stress, atherogenic modifications to LDL, and platelet aggregation: studies in humans and in atherosclerotic apolipoprotein E-deficient mice," Am J Clin Nutr. 2000 May;71(5):1062-76.

The 2000 study provides some interesting history of pomegranate use:

> The pomegranate tree, which is said to have flourished in the garden of Eden, has been used extensively in the folk medicine of many cultures. In ancient Greek mythology, pomegranates were known as the "fruit of the dead" and in the ancient Hebrew tradition, pomegranates adorned the vestments of the high priest. The Babylonians regarded pomegranate seeds as an agent of resurrection, the Persians believed the seeds conferred invincibility on the battlefield, and for the ancient Chinese the seeds symbolized longevity and immortality. Edible parts of pomegranate fruit (about 50% of total fruit weight) comprise 80% juice and 20% seeds. Fresh juice contains 85% water, 10% total sugars, and 1.5% pectin, ascorbic acid, and polyphenolic flavonoids.[10]

A 2005 study published in the *Proceedings of the National Academy of Sciences of the United States of America* notes "that pomegranate fruit extract (PFE) possesses remarkable antitumor-promoting effects" and suggests "that pomegranate juice may have cancer-chemopreventive as well as cancer-chemotherapeutic effects against prostate cancer in humans." [11] Another study conducted by researchers from the University of California, Los Angels, CA and The University of Texas M.D. Anderson Cancer Center, Houston, Texas states, "the polyphenolic phytochemicals in the pomegranate can play an important role in the modulation of inflammatory cell signaling in colon cancer cells."[12] Moreover, there are many more studies on the Heart and blood related benefits of tomatoes, pomegranates, and red wine as well as other red foods.

---

[10] Ibid., p. 1062-76.

[11] Arshi Malik, Farrukh Afaq, Sami Sarfaraz, Vaqar M. Adhami, Deeba N. Syed, and Hasan Mukhtar, "Pomegranate fruit juice for chemoprevention and chemotherapy of prostate cancer," PNAS October 11, 2005 vol. 102 no. 41 14813-14818.

[12] Lynn S. Adams,,, Navindra P. Seeram,, Bharat B. Aggarwal,, Yasunari Takada,, Daniel Sand, and, David Heber, "Pomegranate Juice, Total Pomegranate Ellagitannins, and Punicalagin Suppress Inflammatory Cell Signaling in Colon Cancer Cells," Journal of Agricultural and Food Chemistry 2006 54 (3), 980-985.

Green is for the Liver

Many green foods are cooling, clear Liver fire, and treat high blood pressure due to Yin Xu Yang Kang (yin deficiency with yang uprising).

Celery is cooling, clears Liver fire and is beneficial for the reduction of high blood pressure. Green tea decreases total lipids and cholesterol:

> Tea catechin supplementation increased fecal excretion of total lipids and cholesterol. The results demonstrate that tea catechins exert a hypocholesterolemic effect in cholesterol-fed rats.[13]

The cooling and anti-inflammatory effects of green foods are reflected in research noting that "green tea induces a significant rise in plasma antioxidant activity."[14] The Journal of the National Cancer Institute published the following article on the anticancer properties of green tea:

> Tea consumption in the world is very high and ranks second to water consumption. It is prepared from the dried leaves of Camellia sinensis. Most tea consumed in the world can be classified in two forms, green tea (approximately 20%) and black tea (approximately 80%). Extensive studies from this and other laboratories over the last 10 years have verified cancer chemopreventive effects of a polyphenol mixture derived from green tea against many animal tumor bioassay systems. In these studies, oral consumption or topical application of green tea polyphenols or its major constituent epigallocatechin- 3-gallate has been shown to offer protection against all stages of multistage carcinogenesis that include initiation, promotion, and progression. A study has also shown that green tea consumption can inhibit the growth of established skin papillomas in mice. Epidemiologic studies have not provided conclusive results but tend to suggest that green tea may reduce

---

[13] Muramatsu K, Fukuyo M, Hara Y.; "Effect of green tea catechins on plasma cholesterol level in cholesterol-fed rats," J Nutr Sci Vitaminol (Tokyo). 1986 Dec;32(6):613-22.

[14] LEENEN, ROODENBURG, TIJBURG, WISEMAN, "A single dose of tea with or without milk increases plasma antioxidant activity in humans," European journal of clinical nutrition, 2000, vol. 54, no1, pp. 87-92.

the risk associated with cancers of the bladder, prostate, esophagus, and stomach.[15]

Yellow is for the Spleen

Yellow belongs to the Earth element. Naturally, the Earth promotes many things in the realm of dietetics. Orange or yellow foods benefit the Spleen. This includes carrots, pumpkins, yams, and oranges.

Beta-carotene is a healthy component of foods. It is a red-orange pigment and a precursor to vitamin A. However, large doses of beta-carotene supplementation outside of naturally occurring food sources may increase the risk of lung cancer and may also lead to carotenodermia (orange skin). [16]

White is for the Lung

Bai Mu Er (white mushroom) is most commonly used in food treatments and is seldom used in herbal formulas. To prepare Bai Mu Er, first soak it to make it soft. Next, mix it with chicken soup or cook it with vegetables. Bai Mu Er has little flavor of its own and therefore mixes well with other foods. Bai Mu Er has a general function of benefitting the immune system, which refers to supporting Lung Qi. Bai Mu Er nourishes Lung Yin and is useful to treat a dry cough. White onion and garlic (Da Suan) are other white foods known to benefit the immune system and have both antioxidant and anticancer properties. Gingko (Bai Guo) and daikon are examples of white foods used to treat coughing.

Dark is for the Kidney

Hei Zhi Ma (black sesame) has a strong medicinal benefit for the Kidneys and helps to maintain the dark color of hair. Zhi Mai You (black sesame oil) is used as a cooking oil and has antioxidant

---

[15] Nihal Ahmad, Denise K. Feyes, Rajesh Agarwal and Hasan MukhtarJNCI; "Green Tea Constituent Epigallocatechin-3-Gallate and Induction of Apoptosis and Cell Cycle Arrest in Human Carcinoma Cells," J Natl Cancer Inst (1997) 89 (24): 1881-1886.
[16] Russel, R.M. (2002), "Beta-carotene and lung cancer,". Pure Appl. Chem. 74 (8): 1461–1467.

properties. Other nourishing black foods include black soybean (Hei Dou) and black yam. Black chicken is the chief ingredient in the formula Wu Ji Bai Feng Wan. Eggplant tonifies the Kidneys and invigorates the blood.

Overview

It is healthy to eat meals with a variety of different colors in the daily diet. According to Chinese medicine, the five colors of food enter the five organ systems and impart a spectrum of nourishment to the body.

The Five Tastes

Wood Element: Liver disease

Sour is the taste associated with the Liver. A little sour taste is beneficial and excess sour taste is detrimental to the Liver.

Metal controls Liver Wood and spicy is the taste associated with Metal. Avoid hot spicy foods so that Metal does not over-control Wood.

Metal Element: Lung disease

Fire controls Metal and bitter is the flavor associated with Fire. Avoid excess bitter flavors to avoid over-controlling Metal.

Earth Element: Spleen and Stomach sickness

Avoid sour and sweet flavors for Spleen and Stomach illnesses. Wood controls Earth. Sour is the flavor associated with Wood. Avoid excess sour flavors to avoid over-controlling Earth. From a scientific viewpoint, excess sour foods in the diet may create or aggravate an excess stomach acid disorder.

Sweet is the flavor associated with Earth. Avoid excess sweets to prevent Spleen and Stomach illness.

Fire Element: Heart disease

Avoid salty flavors for Heart disorders so that Water does not over-control Fire. Salty is the flavor of the Water element and Water controls Fire. Modern science commonly supports dietary sodium reduction to help control water and metabolism issues related to heart disease.

Water Element: Kidney disease

Earth controls Kidney Water. Avoid sweet flavors (associated with the Earth element) so that Earth does not over-control Water. Often with Kidney deficiency, especially Kidney Yin deficiency, it is best to avoid sweets. The link between the Water element and western medicine relates with the diagnosis of diabetes.

Chinese Characters for Dietetics

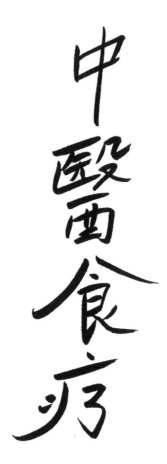

From top to bottom this reads: Chinese, Medicine, Food, Treatment. Medicine, the second character, is a combination of three symbols: arrow, knife or acupuncture needle, and fermentation/alcohol.

Dermatology, Injury, Surgery, Infection

If skin problems are present, after an injury or surgery, or if there is an infection do not eat the following foods:

- Shellfish including shrimp and crab: These foods are particularly contraindicated for psoriasis, eczema and patients with infections. Shellfish tend to turn red when cooked and the concept is that the red from the cooking equates into increased redness and inflammation for these patients. Science confirms that there are several forms of reactions to shellfish including the release of histamines from mast cells.

- Alcohol

- Green onions and chives due to their warming nature are contraindicated.

- Mushrooms and bamboo shoots: They grow too fast and therefore make infections grow too fast also.

- Roasted or barbecued foods: Top contraindications are attributed to roasted duck, goose, and Peking duck.

- Chicken, especially rooster, is contraindicated because it tonifies Yang.

- Goat meat

- Tarot

- Soft drink: Sugar based drinks make infections grow. Also, soft drinks may make changes to the bodily pH thereby contributing to infections.

- Peanuts, especially dry roasted peanuts, are contraindicated.

FDA Industry Guides for Food Labeling

The U.S. Food and Drug Administration (FDA) determines a DV (Daily Value) for healthy food intake for children and adults over four years of age with a total intake of 2,000 calories per day. The table below lists the current DV's issued by the FDA. To calculate the percentage of the DV a particular food or meal contains, divide the amount of the nutrient contained in the food or meal by the DV.

Food Component	DV
Total Fat	65 grams (g)
Saturated Fat	20 g
Cholesterol	300 milligrams (mg)
Sodium	2,400 mg
Potassium	3,500 mg
Total Carbohydrate	300 g
Dietary Fiber	25 g
Protein	50 g
Vitamin A	5,000 International Units (IU)
Vitamin C	60 mg
Calcium	1,000 mg
Iron	18 mg
Vitamin D	400 IU
Vitamin E	30 IU
Vitamin K	80 micrograms µg
Thiamin	1.5 mg
Riboflavin	1.7 mg
Niacin	20 mg
Vitamin B_6	2 mg
Folate	400 µg
Vitamin B_{12}	6 µg
Biotin	300 µg
Pantothenic acid	10 mg
Phosphorus	1,000 mg
Iodine	150 µg
Magnesium	400 mg
Zinc	15 mg
Selenium	70 µg
Copper	2 mg
Manganese	2 mg
Chromium	120 µg
Molybdenum	75 µg
Chloride	3,400 mg

Food Monographs

Cereals

Cereals are edible seeds from grasses and include rice, wheat, spelt, barley, oats, rye, sorghum, millet and corn.

Rice

Long Grain Rice (Geng Mi, Jing Mi, Da Mi)

Southern China and India are known for long grain rice, oryza sativa. Long grain rice is firmer than many forms of rice and is not sticky (non-glutinous). It has a neutral temperature, is sweet, enters the Spleen and Stomach channels and benefits the Spleen and Stomach. Both non-glutinous and glutinous rice are the seeds of the grass Oryza sativa.

Long Grain Brown Rice, cooked		
Source: USDA National Nutrient Database for Standard Reference		
Nutrient	**Units**	**Value per 100 grams**
Proximates		
Water	g	73.09
Energy	kcal	111
Energy	kJ	464
Protein	g	2.58
Total lipid (fat)	g	0.90
Ash	g	0.46
Carbohydrate, by difference	g	22.96
Fiber, total dietary	g	1.8
Sugars, total	g	0.35
Sucrose	g	0.35
Minerals		
Calcium, Ca	mg	10
Iron, Fe	mg	0.42
Magnesium, Mg	mg	43
Phosphorus, P	mg	83

Potassium, K	mg	43
Sodium, Na	mg	5
Zinc, Zn	mg	0.63
Copper, Cu	mg	0.100
Manganese, Mn	mg	0.905
Selenium, Se	mcg	9.8
Vitamins		
Thiamin	mg	0.096
Riboflavin	mg	0.025
Niacin	mg	1.528
Pantothenic acid	mg	0.285
Vitamin B-6	mg	0.145
Folate, total	mcg	4
Choline, total	mg	9.2
Betaine	mg	0.5
Vitamin E (alpha-tocopherol)	mg	0.03
Vitamin K (phylloquinone)	mcg	0.6
Lipids		
Fatty acids, total saturated	g	0.180
Fatty acids, total monounsaturated	g	0.327
Fatty acids, total polyunsaturated	g	0.323
Amino acids		
Tryptophan	g	0.033
Threonine	g	0.095
Isoleucine	g	0.109
Leucine	g	0.214
Lysine	g	0.099
Methionine	g	0.058
Cystine	g	0.031
Phenylalanine	g	0.133
Tyrosine	g	0.097
Valine	g	0.151
Arginine	g	0.196
Histidine	g	0.066
Alanine	g	0.151
Aspartic acid	g	0.242
Glutamic acid	g	0.526
Glycine	g	0.127
Proline	g	0.121
Serine	g	0.134

Medium Grain Rice

Medium grain rice has a neutral temperature and is common in Northern China, Japan, and Korea. It is a little sticky and therefore well suited for sushi preparations.

Medium Grain Brown Rice, cooked		
Source: USDA National Nutrient Database for Standard Reference		
Nutrient	**Units**	**Value per 100 grams**
Proximates		
Water	g	72.96
Energy	kcal	112
Energy	kJ	469
Protein	g	2.32
Total lipid (fat)	g	0.83
Ash	g	0.39
Carbohydrate, by difference	g	23.51
Fiber, total dietary	g	1.8
Minerals		
Calcium, Ca	mg	10
Iron, Fe	mg	0.53
Magnesium, Mg	mg	44
Phosphorus, P	mg	77
Potassium, K	mg	79
Sodium, Na	mg	1
Zinc, Zn	mg	0.62
Copper, Cu	mg	0.081
Manganese, Mn	mg	1.097
Vitamins		
Thiamin	mg	0.102
Riboflavin	mg	0.012
Niacin	mg	1.330
Pantothenic acid	mg	0.392
Vitamin B-6	mg	0.149
Folate, total	mcg	4
Lipids		
Fatty acids, total saturated	g	0.165
Fatty acids, total monounsaturated	g	0.3
Fatty acids, total polyunsaturated	g	0.296
Amino acids		
Tryptophan	g	0.030
Threonine	g	0.085
Isoleucine	g	0.098

Leucine	g	0.191
Lysine	g	0.088
Methionine	g	0.052
Cystine	g	0.028
Phenylalanine	g	0.119
Tyrosine	g	0.087
Valine	g	0.136
Arginine	g	0.175
Histidine	g	0.059
Alanine	g	0.135
Aspartic acid	g	0.217
Glutamic acid	g	0.472
Glycine	g	0.114
Proline	g	0.109
Serine	g	0.120

●Sweet Rice (Glutinous Rice, Nuo Mi, 糯米)

Sweet Rice is a short grain Asian rice that is very sticky and has a warming temperature. It is a glutinous rice. Glutinous implies that sweet rice is sticky, however, rice does not contain gluten. Rice does not contain gluten.

Gluten is a protein composite that is chewy and is in wheat, spelt, barley, and rye. Gluten sensitivity is common and therefore rice is a good choice for those affected by gluten sensitivity.

Glutinous Rice Root (Nuo Dao Gen Xu)

Nuo Dao Gen Xu is astringent, sweet, and neutral. This herb enters the Lung, Liver, and Kidney channels and is useful for the treatment of night sweating and spontaneous sweating.

Wild Rice

There are four species of wild rice. Northern wild rice is indigenous to the US Midwest, another wild rice is native to the Atlantic and Gulf coasts of the US, Texas wild rice is highly endangered and is from the San Marcos River in Texas, and Manchurian wild rice is native to China.

Cooked Wild Rice		
Source: USDA National Nutrient Database for Standard Reference		
Nutrient	**Units**	**Value per 100 grams**
Proximates		
Water	g	73.93
Energy	kcal	101
Energy	kJ	423
Protein	g	3.99
Total lipid (fat)	g	0.34
Ash	g	0.40
Carbohydrate, by difference	g	21.34
Fiber, total dietary	g	1.8
Sugars, total	g	0.73
Sucrose	g	0.33
Glucose (dextrose)	g	0.20
Fructose	g	0.20
Minerals		
Calcium, Ca	mg	3
Iron, Fe	mg	0.60
Magnesium, Mg	mg	32
Phosphorus, P	mg	82
Potassium, K	mg	101
Sodium, Na	mg	3
Zinc, Zn	mg	1.34
Copper, Cu	mg	0.121
Manganese, Mn	mg	0.282
Selenium, Se	mcg	0.8
Vitamins		
Thiamin	mg	0.052
Riboflavin	mg	0.087
Niacin	mg	1.287
Pantothenic acid	mg	0.154
Vitamin B-6	mg	0.135
Folate, total	mcg	26
Choline, total	mg	10.2
Carotene, beta	mcg	2
Vitamin A, IU	IU	3
Lutein + zeaxanthin	mcg	64
Vitamin E (alpha-tocopherol)	mg	0.24
Vitamin K (phylloquinone)	mcg	0.5
Lipids		
Fatty acids, total saturated	g	0.049
Fatty acids, total monounsaturated	g	0.050

Fatty acids, total polyunsaturated	g	0.213
Amino acids		
Tryptophan	g	0.049
Threonine	g	0.127
Isoleucine	g	0.167
Leucine	g	0.276
Lysine	g	0.170
Methionine	g	0.119
Cystine	g	0.047
Phenylalanine	g	0.195
Tyrosine	g	0.169
Valine	g	0.232
Arginine	g	0.308
Histidine	g	0.104
Alanine	g	0.223
Aspartic acid	g	0.384
Glutamic acid	g	0.695
Glycine	g	0.182
Proline	g	0.140
Serine	g	0.211

Brown and White Rice Compared

Brown and white rice have similar amounts of calories, carbohydrates and proteins. In both brown and white rice, the husk is removed. However, white rice has the nutritious inner bran and germ layers removed. Many nutrients are stripped from the rice when making white rice. Enriched white rice involves an industrial process to restore some, but not all, of the removed nutrients.

Black and Red Rice

Black rice is non-glutinous and turns dark purple when cooked. It has a high mineral content, including iron. Research shows that black rice has powerful antioxidant properties.[17] Red rice is a non-glutinous long grain rice with a red colored bran. Studies also

---

[17] Haruyo Ichikawa, Takashi Ichiyanagi, Bing Xu, Yoichi Yoshii, Masaharu Nakajima, Tetsuya Konishi. Journal of Medicinal Food. December 2001, 4(4): 211-218. doi:10.1089/10966200152744481.

show that both black and red rice decrease atherosclerotic plaque formation.[18, 19]

● Red Yeast Rice (Hong Qu Mi)

This herb has been part of the Chinese medicine pharmacopeia since the Tang Dynasty (618-907 CE). It is created by taking rice and fermenting it with a special strain of yeast, monascus purpureus. This process gives the rice its red color. Red yeast rice is not to be confused with red rice, which has a naturally occurring red color to the bran. Hong Qu Mi is sweet, acrid, and warming and enters the Spleen, Liver, and Large Intestine channels. It benefits the Spleen and Stomach, helps with the digestion of food, and invigorates blood circulation.

Hong Qu Mi contains lovastatin. Lovastatin is used in pharmaceutical drugs such as Mevacor, Advicor, Altocor, Altoprev, and Statosan to lower cholesterol. Notably, oyster mushrooms also contain a significant amount of lovastatin. Research concludes that Hong Qu Mi lowers cholesterol.

> Red yeast rice significantly reduces total cholesterol, LDL cholesterol, and total triacylglycerol concentrations compared with placebo and provides a new, novel, food-based approach to lowering cholesterol in the general population.[20]

Administering concentrated doses of red yeast rice in single herb form is not traditional. It is typically combined in formulas with other herbs such as Mai Ya and Shan Zha for digestion issues and Yan Hu Suo and Hong Hua for injuries.

---

[18] Wen Hua Ling, Qi Xuan Cheng, Jing Ma and Tong Wang; "Red and Black Rice Decrease Atherosclerotic Plaque Formation and Increase Antioxidant Status in Rabbits,"
J. Nutr. May 1, 2001 vol. 131 no. 5 1421-1426.
[19] Xiaodong Xia, Wenhua Ling, Jing Ma, Min Xia, Mengjun Hou, Qing Wang, Huilian Zhu and Zhihong Tang; "An Anthocyanin-Rich Extract from Black Rice Enhances Atherosclerotic Plaque Stabilization in Apolipoprotein E–Deficient Mice," J. Nutr. August 1, 2006 vol. 136 no. 8 2220-2225.
[20] David Heber, Ian Yip, Judith M Ashley, David A Elashoff, Robert M Elashoff and Vay Liang W Go; "Cholesterol-lowering effects of a proprietary Chinese red-yeast-rice dietary supplement,"; Am J Clin Nutr February 1999 vol. 69 no. 2 231-236.

Rice Oil

Rice oil has a high smoke point and therefore is a suitable oil for deep frying and stir frying foods.

Gu Ya (Rice Sprout)

Gu Ya enters the Spleen and Stomach channels. It is sweet and neutral. Gu Ya is a commonly used herb to assist digestion and to strengthen the Spleen and Stomach.

Clinical Usage of Rice

Wu Geng Fan (5am Rice Meal)

Wu is five, geng means o'clock and fan is translated as steamed rice or rice meal.

Wu Geng Fan is a dish of rice prepared with a little salt and oil when cooking it. It has a tonifying property due the timing of eating the rice dish. Wake at 5am, eat the rice, then relax and return to bed for additional sleep. Wu Geng Fan is an early breakfast of rice that tonifies Qi and Blood. To complete the restorative process, simply wake from 8 to 9 am.

This is a sleeping schedule combined with a rice breakfast designed for tonification and recuperation. The 5am sunrise time combined with the yang qi of the rice helps the Spleen and Stomach to recover. Benefits are notable after several days. Care must be taken with patients who are overweight due to eating combined with this sleeping schedule.

This is known as an inexpensive way to tonify the body for the poor farmer who is unable to buy chicken. It is also an important dish for those suffering from illness or in the process of recovery. Additionally, this is a traditional preparation to help restore the body after delivering a baby.

Wu Geng Fan may also be used to nourish patients suffering from Wu Geng Xie, 5am diarrhea (Xie is diarrhea). This condition is due to Kidney and Spleen Yang deficiency. It is cold in the morning and therefore the Kidney and Spleen are weaker at this time. This type of diarrhea is watery and loose.

Rice in a formula to help the function or moderate toxicity
Gui Zhi Tang
Gui Zhi Tang is an herbal formula for a deficiency type common cold (Tai Yang Zhong Feng). Congee, rice porridge, tonifies yang qi. After drinking the herbal formula, eat one cup of congee in order to make the function of the formula stronger.

Bai Hu Tang
Bai Hu Tang, White Tiger Decoction, is a very cold formula and may damage the Stomach Qi. Add Geng Mi to the formula to moderate the effects of Shi Gao to protect the Stomach Qi.

Mi Jiang (juice on top of the rice)
Mi Jiang is the made by boiling rice with extra water and skimming the thick rice juice from the top for consumption. This is not congee but is the thick liquid that forms on the top when cooking rice.

Dehydration is a common pediatric concern that often presents with diarrhea, vomiting, and other digestion disorders. Mi Jiang is used to treat and prevent dehydration. Rice milk available in markets is not usually pure Mi Jiang. Packaged rice milk products typically include added ingredients and additional processing.

A western equivalent for the treatment of dehydration is Pedialyte™. This product is recommended by the American Academy of Pediatrics (AAP) and is used to replenish electrolytes. Severe cases of dehydration are treated with an IV drip that includes a mixture of glucose, salt, and other electrolytes.

Yao Cao Mi Fan (pan fried rice with herbs)

Pan frying rice with herbs increases the warming function of the herbs. This can be done with many herbs such as ginseng, Bai Zhu and a variety of fresh herbs. Yao is medicine/herb, cao is fried, mi is rice and fan is contextually translated as cooked.

Example: Add uncooked rice and Bai Zhu to a hot wok and stir. The property of Bai Zhu becomes more drying and Bai Zhu turns to a darker color. This process imparts Bai Zhu with a greater tonify Spleen and warming function. Typically, the rice is discarded but it can be prepared for consumption.

Rice Recipes

Nuo Mi Shan Yao Ju

This dish is traditionally made with sweet rice and Shan Yao (wild mountain yam). However, another rice may be used as a substitute. Soak Shan Yao and sweet rice in water for 1-2 hours. This makes the cooking process easier. Make a congee from this mixture and add herbs such as Gou Qi Zi, Long Yan Rou, Dang Shen, and others as required. This is an excellent choice for children because it is mild and gently treats conditions such Spleen Qi deficiency, malnutrition and loose stool.

Hong Qu Mi (red yeast rice)

Hong is red, Qu is fermented. This rice benefits the Spleen and Stomach and invigorates the blood. In Chinese cuisine, this rice is valued for its color. It is often cooked with meats and imparts a desirable red color. It is also prepared with rice wines and vinegars.

Modern Applications vs. Chinese medicine

Hong Qu Mi can be found in drug stores in concentrated pill form. It is often used for the treatment of high cholesterol when marketed in this form. A principle statin found in read yeast rice is lovastatin – a chemical known to lower cholesterol. In traditional Chinese medicine, however, a single concentrated pill preparation of this herb does not have an historical antecedent. In Chinese medicine and dietetics, it has been used as a garnish rice or in normal dosages within herbal formulas designed to match treatment principles for a differential diagnosis.

Hong Qu Mi in Unfiltered Rice Wine

Hong Qu Nuo Mi Jiu is a dish prepared with sweet rice (nuo mi), white yeast, red yeast and unfiltered rice wine. Mi Jiu is the type of rice wine that is customarily known as a Japanese style sake. Nuo Mi Jiu is unfiltered sake that has a milky white color to it. It is a very sweet variety of rice wine. Adding Hong Qu to this blend creates a red color and imparts anti-cholesterol properties to the beverage.

Mi Tang, Mi Jiang, Zhu You (rice milk)

This is the rice liquid that floats on the surface of rice gruel during the cooking process. Often called rice milk, it tonifies body Yin and fluids in a similar way that Pedialyte™ has hydrating and restorative properties. Zhu You: 'Zhu' refers to rice congee and 'you' refers to oil. Technically, it is not oil. The term 'you' is in reference to the viscous nature of the liquid.

Wu Gu Mi (5 grain rice)

Five ingredients can be mixed to make steamed rice and may include: Hong Mi (red rice), Hei Mi (黑米, black rice), brown rice, Yi Yi Ren and Hong Dou (red bean) or Lu Dou (mung bean). Soak the ingredients overnight and drain the water the next day. Add new water and cook.

White rice, although popular, is not included because it lacks nutrients or requires enrichment to regain nutrients. Polished white rice from Thailand is very popular and easily digested but is nutritionally a poor choice. Soak brown, red, or black rice overnight to make it easy to digest.

Huang Dou (soybean) with brown or dark rice

Use a 1/5 soybean to 4/5 rice proportion to prepare this nutrient rich food. Soak overnight or use a pressure cooker to make the dish soft and easy to digest.

Wheat (Xiao Mai, Little Wheat)

Wheat is the seed of the grass Triticum aestivum and is over 70% carbohydrate and 13% protein. It contains oils, minerals, vitamins and other nutrients. Wheat is sweet and cooling in its raw form but becomes warming when wheat flour is made into bread. As a result, all bread is more warming compared with rice. Wheat enters the Spleen and Heart channels. Oatmeal, barley, and many wheat products have similar properties to xiao mai (also known as Huai Xiao Mai).

Huai Xiao Mai (raw wheat) and fu xiao mai are different parts of the same plant. Fu Xiao Mai is astringent and stops sweating. It is particularly well suited to stopping night sweating. Xiao Mai nourishes the Heart and calms the spirit. Both are sweet, cool, and enter the Heart channel.

Fu Xiao Mai is the unripe wheat seed and it contains a small amount of juice inside. The interior of the seed has not congealed into the mature form and is therefore less dense. As a result, Fu Xiao Mai floats and Huai Xiao Mai does not float. Fu means floating. Xiao Mai is more substantive and therefore has the function of nourishing the Heart Shen and benefitting the Spleen Qi.

Gan Mai Da Zao Tang

The herbal formula Gan Mai Da Zao Tang contains Gan Cao, Fu Xiao Mai and/or Huai Xiao Mai, and Da Zao. This is termed a food treatment formula for dry organ syndrome because it is comprised of licorice, wheat, and smoked date.

Nuo Mi Mai Zhu

This is a congee made from sweet rice (Nuo Mi) and raw wheat (Xiao Mai). This is a food treatment for the Qi and/or Yin deficiency. Other herbs such as Shan Yao can be added to enhance the functions of the formula.

Wheat Sprouts

The raw, germinated wheat sprouts are juiced or even dried into powder form. This is popular in Japan to enhance nutrition and benefit the immune system.

Mai Ya (Barley Sprouts)

Barley and wheat are different grasses from the Poaceae family. Although barley and wheat are similar foods, Mai Ya has distinct characteristics. Mai Ya is sweet, neutral, benefits digestion, restrains lactation, and opens Liver Qi stagnation.

Mai Ya is beneficial for women with breast engorgement. Dry fry 4 lian of mai ya in a wok and then add 2-3 cups of water and boil this herb tea. Drink this tea over a period of several days to restrain lactation.

Wheat flour, whole-grain		
Source: USDA National Nutrient Database for Standard Reference		
Nutrient	**Units**	**Value per 100 grams**
Proximates		
Water	g	10.74
Energy	kcal	340
Energy	kJ	1424
Protein	g	13.21
Total lipid (fat)	g	2.50
Ash	g	1.58
Carbohydrate, by difference	g	71.97
Fiber, total dietary	g	10.7
Sugars, total	g	0.41
Sucrose	g	0.36
Glucose (dextrose)	g	0.00
Fructose	g	0.05
Starch	g	57.77
Minerals		
Calcium, Ca	mg	34
Iron, Fe	mg	3.60
Magnesium, Mg	mg	137
Phosphorus, P	mg	357
Potassium, K	mg	363

Sodium, Na	mg	2
Zinc, Zn	mg	2.60
Copper, Cu	mg	0.410
Manganese, Mn	mg	4.067
Selenium, Se	mcg	61.8
Vitamins		
Thiamin	mg	0.502
Riboflavin	mg	0.165
Niacin	mg	4.957
Pantothenic acid	mg	0.603
Vitamin B-6	mg	0.407
Folate, total	mcg	44
Choline, total	mg	31.2
Betaine	mg	72.8
Carotene, beta	mcg	5
Vitamin A, IU	IU	9
Lutein + zeaxanthin	mcg	220
Vitamin E (alpha-tocopherol)	mg	0.71
Tocopherol, beta	mg	0.23
Tocopherol, gamma	mg	1.91
Vitamin K (phylloquinone)	mcg	1.9
Lipids		
Fatty acids, total saturated	g	0.430
Fatty acids, total monounsaturated	g	0.283
Fatty acids, total polyunsaturated	g	1.167
Amino acids		
Tryptophan	g	0.174
Threonine	g	0.367
Isoleucine	g	0.443
Leucine	g	0.898
Lysine	g	0.359
Methionine	g	0.228
Cystine	g	0.275
Phenylalanine	g	0.682
Tyrosine	g	0.275
Valine	g	0.564
Arginine	g	0.648
Histidine	g	0.357
Alanine	g	0.489
Aspartic acid	g	0.722
Glutamic acid	g	4.328
Glycine	g	0.569
Proline	g	2.075
Serine	g	0.620

Celiac Disease and Gluten

Celiac disease is an intolerance to gluten. Gluten is in wheat, rye, spelt and barley. Celiac disease affects over 1% of people in the USA. Gluten is a protein composite that is chewy and gives dough its elasticity. For those with celiac disease, ingestion of gluten triggers an autoimmune reaction that damages the small intestine's villi thereby preventing them from absorbing nutrients.

Celiac disease, also known as nontropical sprue, is an autoimmune disorder of the small intestine characterized by a variety of symptoms that may include diarrhea, constipation, nausea and vomiting, fatigue, abdominal bloating, weakness, bone pain, weight loss and malnutrition. The stool may float, contain blood or may be excessively foul smelling. Celiac disease is asymptomatic in some instances.

If those with the intolerance continue to eat gluten, studies show a significant increase in the risk for gastrointestinal cancer. All rice (including glutinous rice), millet, amaranth and quinoa do not contain gluten and are therefore healthy choices for those on a gluten free diet.

Oats contain avenin, a glutinous protein similar to gluten found in wheat. Oats processed near wheat facilities may be cross-contaminated with wheat gluten. As a result, there is controversy regarding the use of oats in a gluten free diet. However, studies show that oats are tolerated by those with celiac. [21] Some medications contain gluten. For those with celiac disease, a gluten free diet allows the villi of the small intestine to heal.

A positive blood test for the antibodies tGA (antitissue transglutaminase antibody) or EMA (anti-endomysium antibody) are indicators that there is an intolerance to gluten. If positive, a biopsy of the small intestine may be taken to look for atrophy of the villi.

---

[21] Janatuinen EK, Kemppainen TA, Pikkarainen PH, et al. (March 2000). "Lack of cellular and humoral immunological responses to oats in adults with coeliac disease."

Corn (Yu Mi)

Yu is translated as jade and mi is rice – 'Jade Rice'. Corn, a grass of the zea mays family, originated in what is now Central America and Mexico. It was cultivated by prehistoric indigenous peoples and later by the Aztecs and Mayans. Corn is a major crop in the USA and has food, feed and industrial uses. The USDA (United States Department of Agriculture) notes that corn is the primary feed grain in the USA, accounting for more than 90 percent of total feed grain production and use. In the USA, corn averages over 85 million planted acres per year and yields over 150 million bushels of corn. Corn oil is valued for its high smoke point, making it a good choice for frying foods.

The food portion of corn is the fresh or dried seed, which is bland, sweet and neutral. Corn enters the Lung and Stomach channels and promotes urination.

Yu Mi Xu (Corn Silk)

Yu Mi Xu is sweet, bland, and neutral and enters the Urination Bladder, Liver and Kidney channels. Yu Mi Xu is used to treat edema, dysuria, and damp-heat in the Live and Gallbladder.

Corn Soup for Cough

Use fresh or dried Yu Mi Xu or the entire ear of corn (corn silk, ear leaves, kernels, husks, and stem). Add Chen Pi and Dong Gua (winter melon). Use either candied winter melon or fresh winter melon. This soup promotes urination and is useful to soothe a cough. It is flavorful and therefore easy to administer to children.

Corn Soup for Edema

Take Yu Mi Xu or the entire fresh ear of corn and add Shan Yao and Chi Shao Dou. Drink the soup and eat the ingredients. This soup promotes urination and is beneficial for patients with Spleen Qi deficiency, Kidney disorders, and edema. This soup is a good choice for diabetics.

Corn, yellow		
Source: USDA National Nutrient Database for Standard Reference		
Nutrient	**Units**	**Value per 100 grams**
Proximates		
Water	g	10.37
Energy	kcal	365
Energy	kJ	1527
Protein	g	9.42
Total lipid (fat)	g	4.74
Ash	g	1.20
Carbohydrate, by difference	g	74.26
Fiber, total dietary	g	7.3
Sugars, total	g	0.64
Minerals		
Calcium, Ca	mg	7
Iron, Fe	mg	2.71
Magnesium, Mg	mg	127
Phosphorus, P	mg	210
Potassium, K	mg	287
Sodium, Na	mg	35
Zinc, Zn	mg	2.21
Copper, Cu	mg	0.314
Manganese, Mn	mg	0.485
Selenium, Se	mcg	15.5
Vitamins		
Thiamin	mg	0.385
Riboflavin	mg	0.201
Niacin	mg	3.627
Pantothenic acid	mg	0.424
Vitamin B-6	mg	0.622
Folate, total	mcg	19
Vitamin A, RAE	mcg_RAE	11
Carotene, beta	mcg	97
Carotene, alpha	mcg	63
Vitamin A, IU	IU	214
Lutein + zeaxanthin	mcg	1355
Vitamin E (alpha-tocopherol)	mg	0.49
Vitamin K (phylloquinone)	mcg	0.3
Lipids		
Fatty acids, total saturated	g	0.667
Fatty acids, total monounsaturated	g	1.251
Fatty acids, total polyunsaturated	g	2.163

Amino acids		
Tryptophan	g	0.067
Threonine	g	0.354
Isoleucine	g	0.337
Leucine	g	1.155
Lysine	g	0.265
Methionine	g	0.197
Cystine	g	0.170
Phenylalanine	g	0.463
Tyrosine	g	0.383
Valine	g	0.477
Arginine	g	0.470
Histidine	g	0.287
Alanine	g	0.705
Aspartic acid	g	0.655
Glutamic acid	g	1.768
Glycine	g	0.386
Proline	g	0.822
Serine	g	0.447

Yi Yi Ren (Job's tears, Coix seeds, Pearl Barley)

Yi Yi Ren is sweet, bland, and cooling. It enters the Spleen, Lung, and Kidney channels. This herbal medicine is now available in some supermarkets and is often labeled pearl barely. Yi Yi Ren promotes urination to drain dampness, treats wind damp bi pain, and has a special function to benefit the skin.

Nou Mi Ji (sake, rice wine) can be combined with Yi Yi Ren. When combined, the nou Mi Jiu is especially useful for treating the cold type of arthritis pain that is worse in the winter. The patient may drink the wine and can eat the Yi Yi Ren. In some preparations, the Yi Yi Ren is powdered and then added to the wine.

Tubers

Potato, Sweet Potato, and Shan Yao

The potato is sweet and neutral. It enters the Spleen and Stomach channels. The sweet potato is sweet and neutral. It enters the Spleen, Kidney, Large Intestine, and Stomach channels.

Native to Mexico and South America, the potato is now grown worldwide including large production in the USA and China. Potatoes regulate bowel movements and are beneficial to patients with gastroenteritis or stomach ulcers. Potatoes have a significant fiber content, which eases bowel movements. However, the medicinal function of potatoes is very mild. Potatoes are a healthy food choice more than a medicine.

Sweet potatoes may have either white or orange flesh. Sweet potatoes are from the Convolvulaceae family and are distinct from yams, which are from the Dioscoreae family, although they share many properties. The herb Shan Yao is from the Dioscoreae family and is sweet and neutral. It enters the Kidney, Lung, and Spleen channels. Shan Yao tonifies the Qi of the Spleen, Stomach, and Lungs. This yam also tonifies Lung and Kidney Yin. Shan Yao has the special function of treating Wasting and Thirsting Syndrome and is beneficial for diabetics.

Shan Yao and sweet potatoes have properties that lower cholesterol.[22] Also, both contain DHEA (dehydroepiandrosterone). DHEA is a naturally occurring steroid hormone that is produced by humans, primarily in the adrenal glands and gonads. DHAE is a cortisol agonist and has anti-depressant effects.[23, 24] Sweet potatoes with a deep orange color are good sources of beta-carotene.

---

[22] In Suk SON, Ji Hyun KIM, Ho Yong SOHN, Kun Ho SON, Jong-Sang KIM and Chong-Suk KWON, "Antioxidative and Hypolipidemic Effects of Diosgenin, a Steroidal Saponin of Yam (Dioscorea spp.), on High-Cholesterol Fed Rats", Biosci. Biotechnol. Biochem., Vol. 71, 3063-3071 (2007) .

[23] O. Hechter, A. Grossman and R.T. Chatterton Jr (1887). "Relationship of dehydroepiandrosterone and cortisol in disease". *Medical Hypotheses* 49: 85-91.

[24] Peter Gallagher BSc(Hons) and Allan Young MB, ChB, MPhil, Ph.D, MRCPsych (2002). "Cortisol/DHEA Ratios in Depression". Neuropsychopharmacology 26.

Potatoes and yams are rich in potassium, vitamin C, manganese and vitamin B6. They are a beneficial food for those with high blood pressure due to potassium deficiency.

Juice can be made from potatoes or sweet potatoes. Juice the potatoes in a juice machine, then, add honey and drink. This is particularly beneficial if taken in the morning as a means to line, soothe and protect the stomach. Sweet potatoes can be added to rice to make congee. Initially, the Chinese grew sweet potatoes as means to produce a crop in difficult soil conditions. It was added to rice and eventually became accepted as a quality food combination. Later, sweet potatoes were discovered to be a healthy food choice to lower the incidence of colon cancer.[25, 26] Sweet potato leaf is often available in Asian-style supermarkets. This vegetable has healthy antioxidant properties.[27] It is considered a healthy food choice for diabetics.

---

[25] Yanjun Zhang, Shaiju K. Vareed and Muraleedharan G. Nair. "Human tumor cell growth inhibition by nontoxic anthocyanidins, the pigments in fruits and vegetables". Life Sciences, Volume 76, Issue 13, 11 February 2005, pp 1465-1472.

[26] Isselmou Ould Rabah, De-Xing Hou, Shuh-Ichi Komine, and Makoto Fujii. "Potential Chemopreventive Properties of Extract from Baked Sweet Potato (Ipomoea batatas Lam. Cv. Koganesengan)." J. Agric. Food Chem., 2004, 52 (23), pp 7152–7157.

[27] Chang WH, Chen CM, Hu SP, Kan NW, Chiu CC, Liu JF. "Effect of purple sweet potato leaf consumption on the modulation of the antioxidative status in basketball players during training." Asia Pac J Clin Nutr. 2007;16(3):455-61.

Oils

Mechanical Extraction

Expeller pressing is a method for extracting oil using mechanical pressure. Cold pressed oil is expeller pressed below approximately 120 degrees F.

Chemical Extraction

Chemical extraction involves a process by which solvent extraction and oil desolventizing are performed. Solvent extraction uses the petroleum product hexane to remove the oil. Desolventizing the oil involves evaporating the hexane from the extracted oil for reuse. Residual hexane is removed from the extracted oil using mineral oils. According to the EPA (Environmental Protection Agency), some residual hexane remains in the oil.[28] The EPA also documents that hazardous emissions result from the chemical extraction process due to using "hexane, which is classified as a hazardous air pollutant."[29]

Hydrogenated and Partially Hydrogenated Oils

Trans-fatty acids are formed when vegetable oils undergo the industrial process of hydrogenation. Trans fats raise LDL cholesterol levels and increase the risk of coronary heart disease.[30]

Smoke Point

This refers to the temperature at which oils and fats produce smoke and indicates that decomposition of the oil is occurring. Smoking oil undergoes flavor changes, the nutritional value is altered, and carcinogens may be produced.

Refined oils have higher smoke points. In some cases, chemical processes are used to refine oils. *Extra-virgin* oils are made from the first expeller pressing and have the lowest smoke points. *Fine virgin*

---

[28] EPA.gov . AP-42, CH 9.11.1-8: Vegetable Oil Processing, Emissions and Controls, 11/95, http://www.epa.gov/ttnchie1/ap42/ch09/final/c9s11-1.pdf . Retrieved 1-6-2011.
[29] Ibid., 9.11.1.8.
[30] Food and nutrition board, institute of medicine of the national academies (2005). Dietary Reference Intakes for Energy, Carbohydrate, Fiber, Fat, Fatty Acids, Cholesterol, Protein, and Amino Acids (Macronutrients). National Academies Press. p. 423.

oils are made from the second pressing and *pure oil* is a term that refers to a blend of refined and virgin oil.

Smoke points vary greatly dependent upon the specific process used to extract the oil. As a result, the following smoke point information may vary. Oils with high smoke points include the following *refined* oils: rice bran, avocado, safflower, sunflower, sesame, almond. Rice oil is used for deep frying and stir frying throughout China. High smoke point oils may be used for frying. Medium smoke point oils include the following *refined* oils: tea seed (Camellia oleifera, Camellia sinensis or Camellia japonica), canola, grapeseed, soy, coconut, walnut, peanut, sesame. Medium smoke point oils may be used for sautéing and baking. Oils with relatively low smoke points are the following *unrefined* oils: sesame, toasted sesame, corn, coconut, peanut, olive. Flax oil has a very low smoke point and is used as a dressing or sauce but is typically not heated.

Sesame Oil

Sesame oil has a healthy balance of polyunsaturated fats and monounsaturated fats. It is frequently used for stir frying.

Black Sesame

Zhi Mai You (black sesame oil) is often used as a cooking oil and has a stronger medicinal effect than white sesame. Hei Zhi Ma (black sesame seed) benefits the Kidneys and helps to maintain the dark color of hair.

Sesame Paste

Sesame is also made into a paste and combined with walnuts. The combined paste is then mixed with hot water into a creamy cereal.

Sesame Oil Food Treatments

For the treatment of constipation, mix sesame oil with honey and drink the mixture. This is especially helpful for mothers after the delivery of a baby where there has been blood and Yin loss.

A mixture of Chinese medicine sinus related herbs with sesame oil is used for nose oil drops. Mix Bing Pian, Xin Yi Hua and Cang Er Zi with sesame oil to formulate the nose drops.

Sesame oil may be used topically to treat dry, cracking skin. Black sesame oil is more effective. The darker oil has a stronger function.

Olive Oil

Olive oil has a significant concentration of oleic acid, an omega-9 monounsaturated fat. It is known to reduce harmful LDL cholesterol levels while increasing beneficial HDL cholesterol levels. Oleic acid is at least partially responsible for olive oil's ability to lower blood pressure.[31] It is used as a dressing and in low heat applications due to its low smoke point.

Tea Seed Oil (Cha Zi You)

Cha is translated as tea, zi is seed and you is oil. Tea seed oil is not tea tree oil. Tea tree oil, which is melaleuca oil from Australia, is an entirely different substance. Tea seed oil is added to salads and over steamed vegetables after the cooking process. Refined tea seed oil can be processed to have a high smoke point. It is commonly used for stir frying in Hunan Province, China and for frying tempura in Japanese cooking. Tea oil has natural antioxidant properties.[32] Like olive oil, it has a high oleic acid content.

Rice Bran Oil

This oil has a very high smoke point making it useful for stir frying and deep frying. It has a variety of monounsaturated, polyunsaturated, and saturated fats. Rice bran oil has a significant amount of vitamin E and contains vitamin K. Rice bran oil is a rich

---

[31] Terés, S; Barceló-Coblijn, G; Benet, M; Alvarez, R; Bressani, R; Halver, Je; Escribá, Pv (September 2008). "Oleic acid content is responsible for the reduction in blood pressure induced by olive oil". Proceedings of the National Academy of Sciences of the United States of America 105 (37): 13811–6.

[32] Mohammad Ali Sahari, Davood Ataii and Manuchehr Hamedi. "Characteristics of tea seed oil in comparison with sunflower and olive oils and its effect as a natural antioxidant." JOURNAL OF THE AMERICAN OIL CHEMISTS' SOCIETY, Volume 81, Number 6, 585-588, DOI: 10.1007/s11746-006-0945-0.

source of tocotrienols (TRF), a component of vitamin E that is associated with lowering LDL cholesterol.[33]

Soybean Oil

Soybean oil is hot, pungent, and sweet. Soybean oil lubricates the Large Intestine. Soybean oil contains a significant quantity of phytosterols, which have been linked to lowering LDL cholesterol levels.[34] Sources for soybean oil are naturally occurring soybeans and transgenic soybeans. Transgenic soybeans are genetically engineered by inserting genes from an external source into the soybean. Naturally occurring soybeans are often hybridized to enhance specific attributes.

Many foods undergo genetic engineering and/or hybridization. In general, these processes alter properties such as yield, nutritional value, flavor, color and the shelf life of foods.

---

[33] University of Rochester Medical Center (2005, May 12). Can Rice Bran Oil Melt Away Cholesterol?. ScienceDaily. Retrieved January 6, 2011, from http://www.sciencedaily.com /releases/2005/05/050512110703.htm .

[34] Oksana A Matvienko, Douglas S Lewis, Mike Swanson, Beth Arndt, David L Rainwater, Jeanne Stewart and D Lee Alekel. "A single daily dose of soybean phytosterols in ground beef decreases serum total cholesterol and LDL cholesterol in young, mildly hypercholesterolemic men." Am J Clin Nutr July 2002 vol. 76 no. 1 57-64.

Condiments and Liquor

•Yi Tang (Maltose, Barley Malt Sugar)

Yi Tang is the syrup made by combining barley malt with rice powder, however, some preparations use wheat powder instead. It is sweet and slightly warm. Yi Tang enters the Lung, Spleen, and Stomach channels. Yi Tang tonifies the Spleen and Stomach Qi and alleviates abdominal pain due to cold and deficiency. Yi Tang moistens the lungs to stop coughing. It is contraindicated in cases of damp-heat.

•Hong Tang (Red Sugar)

Red sugar is crystallized from squeezed sugarcane juice. Unlike processed white sugar (table sugar), it has not been stripped of minerals and other nutrients. Table sugar not only lacks nutritional value but it also becomes more damp due to processing. Hong Tang is sweet, warm and tonifies Qi. It is used in food treatments for patients with deficiency and cold. To benefit the elderly, Hong Tang is often cooked with chicken.

The formula Jiang Cong Tang is used for the treatment of wind-cold common cold and cold-type stomach pain. Boil Sheng Jiang (fresh ginger), Cong Bai (green onion) and Hong Tang in water.

•Fresh Cane Juice

Fresh cane juice is sweet and very cooling. Once it has been crystallized into Hong Tang, it becomes warming. Fresh cane juice is sold on the streets of China, Thailand and Vietnam. In Vietnam, it is also available in restaurants. It is used for palpitations and/or thirst due to heat exposure in the summer. Cane juice is also canned and sold in stores.

•Bing Tang (Rock Sugar, Ice Sugar)

Made from refined sugarcane juice, it is hardened into large crystals. It is cool, sweet and enters the Lung, Spleen and Stomach channels. Rock sugar moistens and cools the Lungs and is used to treat dry-heat coughs. Rock sugar mildly tonifies Spleen and Stomach Qi.

- Bing Tang is often prepared with Asian pears to nourish Lung Yin.

- The formula Yin Er Bing Tang is used to tonify Yin. Soak Bai Mu Er (Yin Er, white fungus) in water to soften. Later, heat the mixture and add Bing Tang. Eat the Bai Mu Er and drink the soup. Lian Zi (lotus seed) can be added during the preparation.

Honey (Feng Mi, Mi Tang)

Honey is sweet and enters the Lung, Spleen and Large Intestine channels. The temperature of honey varies with the nature of the nectar that it has been derived. Honey may be warming as in the case of lychee honey, neutral when derived from oranges and cooling when derived from alfalfa.

Honey moistens the Lungs to stop coughing and lubricates the Large Intestine to treat constipation. Honey has a very mild function to tonify the Spleen and Stomach Qi. Compared with Yi Tang, honey has less of a tonify Qi function but has a stronger function to lubricate Yin. Honey may cause infant botulism, a rare form of food poisoning, and is not to be given to children under 1 year of age.

Honey is commonly added to herbal powders to make pills and cough related herbs to make syrups. For cough and dry throat:

- Chuan Bei Pi Pa Gao cough syrup's main ingredient is honey.
- Mix Chuan Bei Mu powder with honey and hot water for the treatment of coughs.
- The Pi Pa (loquat) tree is indigenous to southeastern China. An easy home remedy for dry throat with coughing is to combine loquat fruit with honey and mint. Additional herbs can be added to the mixture to enhance the therapeutic value.

- Honey with Bo He (peppermint) and lemon or lime juice is often soothing for sore throats.

Honey lubricates the Large Intestine and moistens dry stool. For deficiency type constipation:

- Eat two raw walnuts and drink a mixture of honey and water prior to sleeping. This is especially helpful for the elderly.
- Mix black sesame (Hei Zhi Ma) powder, finely ground flax seed (Hu Ma Ren) and honey. Hei Zhi Ma has the added benefit of tonifying the Kidneys and darkening the hair.

Children over the age of one year may take 2-3 teaspoons of honey before sleep to relieve bedwetting.

Topically apply honey to canker sores, mouth ulcers, and slow healing ulcerations to soothe the burning sensation.

Royal Jelly

Royal Jelly is a honeybee glandular secretion used to feed larvae in the colony. Bees feed larger quantities of royal jelly to larvae to induce queen bee morphology. Royal Jelly may cause allergic reactions in some humans but may also suppress allergic reactions in others.[35] Royal Jelly may have therapeutic value in the treatment of Grave's disease.[36] It also has been shown to have anti-tumor properties.[37]

Salt (Sea Salt, Natural Salt)

Salt is cold and enters the Kidney, Stomach, and Large Intestine channels. A channel leading mineral, salt leads other herbs and foods to the Kidney channel. It is medicinally used both internally

---

[35] Hideki Oka, Yutaka Emoria, Naomi Kobayashia, Yoshiro Hayashia and Kikuo Nomotob. "Suppression of allergic reactions by royal jelly in association with the restoration of macrophage function and the improvement of Th1/Th2 cell responses." International Immunopharmacology
Volume 1, Issue 3, March 2001, Pages 521-532.

[36] Cihangir Erem, Orhan Deger, Ercüment Ovali and Yasam Barlak. "The effects of royal jelly on autoimmunity in Graves' disease." ENDOCRINE, Volume 30, Number 2, 175-183.

[37] Tamura T, Fujii A, Kuboyama N. "Antitumor effects of royal jelly (RJ)." Nippon Yakurigaku Zasshi. 1987 Feb;89(2):73-80.

and topically. Excess salt intake exacerbates high blood pressure and edema. Deficient salt intake can lead to electrolyte imbalances.

Internal Usage

- The herbal formula Liu Wei Di Huang Tang often has a little salt added to lead the herbs to the Kidney. When taking the herbal pill form of this formula, one can drink warm water with a little bit of salt in it to increase the function of benefitting the Kidneys.

- Cooking chicken with salt tonifies the Kidneys.

Teeth and Gums

- Salt enters the Stomach and Kidney channels and is therefore tooth and gum related. It is cooling and is an effective mouth rinse when mixed into water for the treatment of Stomach Fire or Kidney Yin deficiency teeth infections. Salt may also be added to internal usage herbal formulas for this application.

- Salt is especially good for treating chronic gum diseases due to its antibiotic properties. For periodontal gum pocket disorders, mix salt, baking soda, and hydrogen peroxide and place it directly into the gum pocket. The initial application of the mixture may be painful or irritating.

Heat Therapy

Salt is used to radiate infrared heat. Course salt is better than small, refined grains.

- Dry fry salt in a wok. Next, place the salt in a cheesecloth and place on the affected painful area such as the lower back.

- Fill the navel with salt and use moxa on the top of the salt mound.

Refined Table Salt

Many refined salts, including those made from sea salt and rock salt (mined underground), have anticaking agents added such as sodium silicoaluminate, magnesium carbonate, sodium ferrocyanide, silicon dioxide, or calcium silicate. Refined salt is often heat-blasted and chemically treated, which may strip minerals from the salt. Iodine is often added to salt to enrich the diet.

Vinegar

●Vinegar is sour, warming, and enters the Stomach and Liver channels. Vinegar invigorates the blood and relieves toxicity. Chinese rice vinegar is made by a process of fermenting yeast with rice.

Topical Uses

Vinegar is added to herbs to make an external use paste. Vinegar enhances the blood invigorating function and helps the herbs to penetrate the surface. Examples:

- Lu Shen Wan pills are crushed, mixed with vinegar to form a paste and applied topically to infections.

- Yu Nan Bai Yao powder is mixed with vinegar and applied to external injuries.

Vinegar Softens the Hard

Modern research notes that vinegar is effective in the treatment of arteriole sclerosis. In this condition, the pulse can become excess and wiry due to the tension of the vessel lining when cholesterol hardening makes the vessels firmer. Vinegar is especially effective for heart conditions including angina pain and benefitting the vessels during recovery from a myocardial infarction.

Vinegar and Digestion

Vinegar benefits digestion in small quantities when taken with food. Excess vinegar intake may hurt the stomach or exacerbate stomach ulcers and it is therefore advisable not to drink straight vinegar. Combining vinegar with food prevents unwanted side effects.

It is traditional to add vinegar to noodles and pot stickers and this assists digestion. Also, beans or peanuts pickled in vinegar are part of a traditional breakfast.

Pickled Soybean Recipe

Ingredients
- Sweet black rice vinegar 1 pound
- Regular vinegar   1 pound
- Roasted soybeans   1 pound

Soak the soybeans in the liquid for approximately one week. This is referred to as "Pickled Soybeans." It has a spongy texture and is known for lowering cholesterol. If the flavor is too sour, add a little honey.

Regular vinegar is very sour but tien chu (tien is sweet, chu is vinegar) sweet black rice vinegar is sweet, less sour, and has a more robust flavor.

Postpartum Vinegar Recipe

Ingredients
- Hard boiled egg (no shell)
- Copious amounts of fresh ginger
- Pig feet (gelatin and soft bone)
- Sweet black rice vinegar

This dish is traditionally served to women in the time following the delivery of a baby and is culturally a celebratory dish shared with guests one month after delivery. The dish is not very sour and is hot and spicy with its generous amounts of ginger. It has a mild blood invigorating function. It also tonifies and expels wind.

Pickled Egg

Wash a raw egg in water. Soak the egg in vinegar for two days. Vinegar dissolves the shell but a soft lining remains. Next, poke the egg to let the ingredients flow into the vinegar. Drink the vinegar-egg liquid. This has a similar function to the pickled soybean recipe.

•Alcohol (Jiu)

Alcohol is spicy, bitter, sweet, warm, and slightly toxic. It enters the Heart, Liver, and Stomach channels. Alcohol warms the body, has an uprising and spreading function, tonifies Yang and invigorates blood.

Virtually every culture throughout history has used alcohol. The Chinese character for medicine contains the symbols for alcohol, an arrow, and a needle or knife. This character implies that alcohol is a tool for medicinal purposes. European history is known for the development of grape based alcohols whereas Chinese dietetics is concerned primarily with rice alcohol (Mi Jiu).

Research indicates that red wine may prevent heart disease, in part, due to the fact that "red wines strongly inhibit the synthesis of endothelin-1, a vasoactive peptide that is crucial in the development of coronary atherosclerosis."[38] In Chinese medicine, this relates to the red wine's ability to prevent blood stagnation. Excess alcohol intake is toxic and addictive.

There are many forms of medical alcohols (Yao Jiu). Tonify Kidney Yang herbs are often combined with ginseng and/or Lu Rong and then soaked in alcohol. Alcohol's ability to move through the channels enhances the effects of snakes, Hu Gu (tiger bone)[39], Mu Gua, Du Zhong, and similar herbs for the treatment of wind-damp-bi-pain. Alcohol is widely used in herbal formulas for the treatment of trauma such as bone fractures, bruises, and sprains. These die da formulas are designed for internal use and/or external application. Common herbs for the treatment of injury include san qi, Dang Gui, and many of the invigorate blood category herbs. In many cases, herbs are soaked for one month prior to use. The alcoholic content of herbal liquors must be approximately 40% or higher to stabilize the effectiveness of the herbs and to prevent spoilage.

---

[38] Roger Corder, Julie A. Douthwaite, Delphine M. Lees, Noorafza Q. Khan, Ana Carolina Viseu dos Santos, Elizabeth G. Wood & Martin J. Carrier. "Health: Endothelin-1 synthesis reduced by red wine." Nature 414, 863-864 (20 December 2001).

[39] Tigers are an endangered species and the use of hu gu is illegal in many countries. Poaching and habitat encroachment are major contributors to the depletion of tiger populations.

Beans

Huang Dou (Soybean, "Yellow Bean")

Soybeans have been cultivated in China for thousands of years and are consumed in a variety of forms including tofu, soybean oil, soy sauce, fermented beans, sprouts, and soymilk. The USA is the largest producer of soybeans (over 80 metric tons annually) followed by Brazil, Argentina, and China. Over 90% of US soybean is genetically modified.

Yellow soybean is neutral and sweet. Yellow soybean tonifies the Spleen, benefits the intestines and eliminates tissue fluids for the treatment of edema. According to five element theory, yellow soybean is particularly beneficial to the Spleen because the color yellow and the Spleen belong to the earth element. Black soybeans are similar but also benefit the Kidneys and invigorate the blood. Soybean oil is hot, pungent, and sweet. Soybean oil lubricates the Large Intestine. Soy sauce benefits digestion and may be used externally for the treatment of burns.

Tofu (Bean Curd)

Tofu has been produced in China since the Han Dynasty approximately 2,000 years ago. Tofu later became part of Japanese, Korean, Vietnamese, and Indonesian cuisine. Tofu is cool and sweet. Tofu benefits the Spleen, Stomach, and Large Intestine. Tofu benefits Qi, produces fluids, and cools heat toxins. Tofu may be cooked with vinegar and consumed to treat chronic diarrhea. Tofu is high in protein, relatively low in calories, contains iron, and when traditionally prepared is a significant source of calcium.

Tofu is the curd produced from coagulated soymilk. Shi Gao, gypsum, is the traditional coagulant used in bean curd production and it accounts for the high calcium content in tofu and the cooling temperature as well. Non-traditional coagulants are often used in tofu manufacturing such as magnesium chloride, calcium chloride, vinegar, citric acid, and glucono delta-lactone. However, these replacements for Shi Gao alter the medicinal function of the tofu.

Tofu is produced first by soaking soybeans in water overnight. Next, the soybeans are combined with a little bit of water and run through a juicing machine. The end result is a juice and a fibrous substance. The fiber can be cooked and eaten or used as fertilizer for plants. The raw juice is then filtered but is not yet edible and may cause diarrhea and vomiting if consumed due to a mild toxicity. Next, boil the juice. At this stage, the juice no longer is toxic and is safe for consumption as soymilk. The resultant soymilk has a neutral temperature and has, what is considered by many, an unpleasant scent.

Manufacturers usually employ a chemical process to remove the scent from soymilk and also to alter the flavor. A basic principle of Chinese medicine dietetics is that less processing is better, simple is healthy. In the marketplace, commercial soymilk is usually a healthy food but is processed more than is necessary.

Continue to boil the soymilk and skim off the top layer to make Fu Zhu, a type of noodle, or dry the skimmed layer to make fu pi, tofu skin. Up to this point the tofu products have a neutral temperate. Now, add Shi Gao to the heated soymilk to produce the bean curd. The medicinal temperature of the soymilk has now been changed to cold. A small amount of Shi Gao is added to make soft tofu and a larger amount is added to make hard tofu.

Cooking preparation techniques alter the medicinal temperature of the tofu. For example, deep fried tofu or tofu cooked in chili pepper has a hot medicinal temperature. A shortcut to tofu production is taking soybean powder and cooking it to avoid the need for the juicing process.

Traditional Tofu Cooking Preparations
- Tofu with green vegetables is traditional. Often, cucumber is chosen to enhance the cooling nature of tofu. Cut tofu into small pieces and make a soup with the cucumber and tofu.

- A traditional Japanese preparation is to combine tofu, seaweed, green onion and miso (fermented soybean paste).

- Tofu is often cut into small pieces and presented in a chicken soup with Hai Dai and green onion.

- A beautiful steamed tofu preparation combines tofu with fish, meat, or vegetables. Hollow the center of a brick of tofu and fill it with the ingredients. Place the tofu on a plate and steam the preparation. Garnish with green onion and serve.

External Use of Tofu

- A mixture of soft tofu with cooling herbs such as Huang Bai and Huang Lian may be placed directly on the skin for the treatment of burns, burning sensations, and sunburn.

- A tofu facemask may be made with a mixture of Zhen Zhu (pearl powder) steamed with tofu and other herbs to benefit the skin.

Soybean Sprouts

Da Dou Huang Jian is the name for sun-dried soybean sprouts that literally means big bean yellow curl. It is sweet, neutral and enters the Spleen and Stomach channels. Da Dou Huang Jian has a very mild function of releasing the surface and may be used to clear summer heat with dampness. By comparison, mung bean sprouts are more tender and are smaller at the base than soybean sprouts.

Soy facts

- Soy lecithin and soybean oil intake have been shown to lower cholesterol.[40,41]

---

[40] Thomas A Wilson, Craig M Meservey, Robert J Nicolosi. Soy lecithin reduces plasma lipoprotein cholesterol and early atherogenesis in hypercholesterolemic monkeys and hamsters: beyond linoleate. Atherosclerosis, v140, 1, p147-153, September 1998.
[41] Oksana A Matvienko, Douglas S Lewis, Mike Swanson, Beth Arndt, David L Rainwater, Jeanne Stewart and D Lee Alekel. "A single daily dose of soybean phytosterols in ground beef decreases serum total cholesterol and LDL cholesterol in young, mildly hypercholesterolemic men." Am J Clin Nutr July 2002 vol. 76 no. 1 57-64.

- Lecithin has benefits to the brain, nervous system and can suppress tardive dyskinesia, a neurological disorder characterized by repetitive involuntary movements.[42]

- Eating soy foods has been shown to reduce the risk of prostate cancer.[43]

- Soy foods reduce the risk for osteoporosis and cardiovascular disease.[44]

- Genistein and daidzein are isoflavones, organic compounds that act as phytoestrogens. Soybeans have high concentrations of bioavailable genistein and daidzein. Genistein and daidzein have antitumor and antioxidant properties. [45] Studies show that genistein is both anticarcinogenic and antineoplastic. [46] Genistein and daidzein are also abundant in Ge Gen (kudzu), a popular cooking thickener and Chinese herbal medicine.

- Soy products do not contribute to breast cancer. A study of 18,312 women who previously had breast cancer shows that eating greater than 23 mg of soy per day resulted in greater than a 15% reduction of breast cancer recurrence over women who ate 0.48 mg per day or less. [47] The study

---

[42] Lecithin Can Suppress Tardive Dyskinesia. N Engl J Med 1978; 298:1029-1030.

[43] Marion M. Lee, Scarlett Lin Gomez, Jeffrey S. Chang, Mercy Wey, Run-Tian Wang and Ann W. Hsing. Soy and Isoflavone Consumption in Relation to Prostate Cancer Risk in China. Cancer Epidemiol Biomarkers Prev, July 2003 12; 665.

[44] Scheiber, Michael D. MD, MPH; Liu, James H. MD; Subbiah, M. T.R. PhD; Rebar, Robert W. MD; Setchell, Kenneth D.R. PhD. Dietary inclusion of whole soy foods results in significant reductions in clinical risk factors for osteoporosis and cardiovascular disease in normal postmenopausal women. Menopause, September 2001, v8, 5. p384-392. NAMS Fellowship Findings.

[45] Lori. Coward, Neil C. Barnes, Kenneth D. R. Setchell, Stephen. Barnes. Genistein, daidzein, and their .beta.-glycoside conjugates: antitumor isoflavones in soybean foods from American and Asian diets. J. Agric. Food Chem., 1993, 41 (11), pp 1961–1967.

[46] Wei H, Bowen R, Cai Q, Barnes S, Wang Y. Antioxidant and antipromotional effects of the soybean isoflavone genistein. Department of Environmental Health Sciences, University of Alabama at Birmingham 35294. Proc Soc Exp Biol Med. 1995 Jan;208(1):124-30.

[47] Sarah J. Nechuta1, Bette J. Caan, Wendy Y. Chen, Wei Lu, Zhi Chen, Marilyn L. Kwan, Shirley W. Flatt, Ying Zheng, Wei Zheng, John P. Pierce, Xiao Ou Shu. Vanderbilt University, Nashville, TN; Kaiser Permanente Medical Program, Oakland,

concluded that, "Soy food consumption was not associated with an increased risk of mortality or cancer recurrence among breast cancer survivors." Soy isoflavonoids are referred to as phytoestrogens because they are plant based compounds with estrogenic properties.[48] One theory is that soy isoflavones compete with estrogen for receptor sites and therefore reduce the health risks associated with estrogen.

◆Lu Dou (Mung Bean)

Lu Dou is sweet, cool and enters the Heart and Stomach channels. It clears summer heat and is an antidote for the excess intake of Fu Zi (Radix Aconiti Carmichaeli Praeparata). Lu Dou benefits the skin.

- Lu Dou Gan Cao Tang is prepared by boiling mung beans with sheng gan cao (licorice). This formula is used to relieve toxicity of the body for many applications including chemical poisoning, including excess pesticide exposure.

- Hai Dai Lu Dou Tang is a combination of mung beans with Hai Dai (Thallus Laminariae, seaweed). The mung beans are soaked overnight or boiled until soft. Soak the Hai Dai overnight to soften and then cut into small pieces. Combine the ingredients. This flavorful dish treats Yin deficiency, high blood pressure due to Liver fire, heat-toxin skin disorders, acne, and eczema.

Hei Dou (Black Soybean, Black Bean, Semen Glycine Max)

Hei Dou is sweet, neutral, and enters the Spleen and Kidney channels. Hei Dou is usually roasted and the temperature changes

CA; Harvard University, Boston, MA; Shanghai Center for Disease Control & Prevention, Shanghai, China; University of California-San Diego, San Diego, CA. Postdiagnosis soy food intake and breast cancer survival: Report from the After Breast Cancer Pooling Project. Tuesday, Apr 05, 2011, 1:00 PM - 5:00 PM, Exhibit Hall A4-C, Poster Section 36. American Association for Cancer Research (AACR), 102nd Annual Meeting; Orlando, Florida, USA.

[48] Barnes S. Soy isoflavones--phytoestrogens and what else? J. Nutr. 2004 May;134(5):1225S-1228S.

to warm. It nourishes Kidney Yin and Yang, nourishes the Spleen Qi, and clears dampness and toxins. Similar to yellow soybean, the black color of Hei Dou reflects its special benefits to the Kidney channel.

- A congee is made from combining Hei Dou, Hong Zao (red date, jujube), Nou Mi (sweet rice), Hong Tang (red or brown sugar). This congee is used for the treatment of Kidney Yang deficiency, Spleen Qi deficiency, and sweating and edema of the legs. Although congee is the traditional preparation, a steamed rice preparation of this recipe is effective.

- Hei Dou is conveniently prepped for later use by soaking, steaming, and then refrigerating.

- Dan Dou Chi is an herbal medicine made by fermenting Hei Dou. Dan Dou Chi is used in the treatment of wind-heat conditions. Black bean sauce is made with a salted preparation of Dan Dou Chi. The salted variety is not used in the treatment of wind-heat.

Chi Xiao Dou (Adzuki Bean)

Chi Xiao Dou is sweet, sour, neutral and enters the Heart and Small Intestine channels. Chi Xiao Dou promotes urination to drain dampness. Chi Xiao Dou treats edema, especially when combined with PMS, Leg Qi, obesity, or liver cirrhosis with ascites.

Chi Xiao Dou Li Yu Tang is made with adzuki beans and Li Yu (silver carp fish). Li Yu can be purchased live at Asian markets. To prepare this traditional dish, soak the Chi Xiao Dou overnight. Next, boil the beans until soft with enough water to maintain a broth for soup. Heat a pan or wok with a little oil, ginger and garlic. Add the silver carp fish to brown the skin. Next, add the fish to the bean soup and boil. Eat the Chi Xiao Dou and drink the soup. Eating the fish is optional. Many do not eat the fish because it has many bones. Some choose to put the fish in cheesecloth prior to adding it to the adzuki bean soup.

Tea

Shen Nong, the Divine Farmer, is credited with discovering tea as an antidote to 72 poisons in approximately 200 BCE. Tea is made from the leaves, buds, and internodes of the Camellia sinensis plant. Special preparations may also be made from the twigs of the plant. The tea plant is indigenous to Asia and is typically clipped to form shrubs under two meters in height. The two major varieties are Camellia sinensis sinensis and Camellia sinensis assamica. Camellia sinensis sinensis grows throughout China and reaches a height of up to 3 meters, unclipped. The Assam variety (Camellia sinensis assamica) grows primarily in North-East India, Myanmar, Vietnam, and South China. Assam tea plants reach up to 20 meters in height, unclipped.

Portuguese explorers were introduced to tea in the Macau region in the 1500s. The Portuguese explorers adopted the local pronunciation of tea, later becoming what is now the current English pronunciation of tea. The Mandarin pronunciation of tea is cha.

Tea is bitter and sweet. Green tea is cold or cooling whereas black tea is warming. Tea enters the Heart, Lung, Stomach, Large Intestine, Small Intestine and Urination Bladder channels. Tea clears the upper jiao Shen (spirit) and therefore clears the mind and treats headaches. In the middle jiao, tea benefits the digestion of food and relieves food stagnation. In the lower jiao, tea promotes urination and bowel movements. Green tea's cooling nature makes it suitable for flushing out toxins in cases of urinary tract infections.

Tea is commonly available in white, green, brown, and black preparations. White tea is made from the new buds and young leaves of several varieties of the tea plant. This new growth maintains a silvery white appearance and is a specialty of Fujian province. Green tea, Lu Cha, is made from more mature leaves, buds, and internodes. Green tea and white tea maintain their green and white appearances because the freshly picked tea is steamed or heated and dried to prevent it from withering into a darker color. Steaming or heating the tea inactivates polyphenol oxidase thereby halting the process of oxidation. It is best not to start the day with a cup of green tea prior to eating in order to prevent stomach irritation.

The withering process of tea into darker varieties is due to enzymatic oxidation, however, the term fermentation is often used. Fermentation is an industry term usually referring to oxidation levels and is not related to the chemical process of fermentation. Many refer to green and white tea as unfermented, oolong tea as partially fermented, and black tea as fermented tea.

Brown teas, such as many forms of oolong tea, get their earthy brown color because they are allowed to wither for a longer duration prior to steaming or heating. Tie Guanyin (Ti Kuan Yin) and Dong Ding are popular varieties of oolong tea. Black teas undergo the longest periods of oxidation prior to processing and therefore wither into the darkest colors. Red tea, Hong Cha, is the Chinese term for black tea and is named after the reddish color of tea when consumed as a drink.

English Tea

The English tradition of tea with milk has its origins in Tibet. The Tibetans are known for drinking butter tea (Po Cha, Su You Cha). Butter tea is a combination of tea, yak butter, and salt. This preparation is a high-energy drink that is helpful for Tibetans living at high elevations with cold temperatures and poor growing conditions. The English adapted the tradition of mixing black tea with dairy and added sugar. Adding dairy products and sugar strengthens the warming and tonifying function of the tea. Black tea is warming and is therefore more suitable for colder climates or consumption in the winter. Green tea is cooling and is more suitable for consumption in the summer.

Pu-erh

Pu-erh tea is made from a large leaf variety of Camellia sinensis, primarily grown in the mountains of Yunnan province. It is often pressed into bricks but is also available in loose-leaf form after completing a special process of pressing. The special preparations involved in Pu-erh production allow the tea to mature with age. Unlike other teas, the flavor of pu-erh improves with age.

Pu-erh, like many forms of tea, is known for its antioxidant properties. This is due in part to the presence of catechins and flavonoids in the tea.[49] Pu-erh has the special ability to raise the 'good' HDL cholesterol while lowering levels of the 'bad' LDL cholesterol.[50]

Research shows that pu-erh tea reduces obesity. The study conducted by the Yunnan Provincial Key Laboratory and the College of Food Science and Technology at the Yunnan Agricultural University notes that pu-erh significantly reduced total body weight, adipose pads, LDL cholesterol, and triglycerides.[51] The researchers postulate that the fat reduction may be triggered by pu-erh's ability to boost enzymes such as lipoprotein lipase, hepatic lipase, and hormone sensitive lipase. Pu-erh tea is a traditional compliment to mooncake during the Mooncake Festival (Mid-Autumn Festival). The properties of pu-erh make it well suited to improving digestion when eating oily, fatty, and sweet foods.

Decorative pressed tea ball preparations of pu-erh are made by combining it with Ju Hua (chrysanthemum) or other herbs. The tea balls expand when placed in hot water and often provide a beautiful presentation of the tea. Another special preparation involves cooking the pu-erh inside bamboo to enhance the flavor.

---

[49] Pin-Der Duh, Gow-Chin Yen, Wen-Jye Yen, Bor-Sen Wang, and Lee-Wen Chang. Effects of Pu-erh Tea on Oxidative Damage and Nitric Oxide Scavenging. J. Agric. Food Chem., 2004, 52 (26), pp 8169–8176.

[50] Kuan-Li Kuo, Meng-Shih Weng, Chun-Te Chiang, Yao-Jen Tsai, Shoei-Yn Lin-Shiau, and Jen-Kun Lin. Comparative Studies on the Hypolipidemic and Growth Suppressive Effects of Oolong, Black, Pu-erh, and Green Tea Leaves in Rats. J. Agric. Food Chem., 2005, 53 (2), pp 480–489.

[51] Zhen-Hui Cao, Da-Hai Gu, Qiu-Ye Lin, Zhi-Qiang Xu, Qi-Chao Huang, Hua Rao1, Er-Wei Liu, Jun-Jing Jia, Chang-Rong Ge. Effect of pu-erh tea on body fat and lipid profiles in rats with diet-induced obesity. Phytotherapy Research. Volume 25, Issue 2, pages 234–238, February 2011.

Herbs and Tea

Tea is also a term used in reference to herbal drinks that do not contain any part of the tea plant. Hua Cha, flower tea, is often made from jasmine, chrysanthemum (Ju Hua), and roasted Chinese rosebud (rosa rugosa, Mei Gui Hua).

In Chinese medicine, the opening of flowers is the expression of the free flow of Qi. Consequently, flowers have the general property of treating Liver Qi stagnation. The relationship of flowers and the Liver Qi make flower tea an appropriate match for springtime, the season associated with the Liver.

Jiao Gu Lan (gynostemma pentaphyllum) is a leaf herb that can be prepared as a hot beverage. It is slightly bitter and is often mixed with Gan Cao (licorice) to add sweetness to the flavor. Jiao Gu Lan is often used for its adaptogenic medicinal value. Also, herbal ingredients are often added to tea such as Shan Zha (hawthorn berry) or bitter melon.

Caffeine

The caffeine in tea stimulates the heart and Shen (spirit). As a result, tea increases alertness. However, excessive consumption is over-stimulating. Excessive consumption may induce temporary tachycardia, insomnia or palpitations. Tea is not for everyone as it may cause unwanted side effects.

Fluoride

Tea absorbs fluoride into its leaves. There are approximately 0.5 to 9 mg of fluoride per liter of tea. Excessive tea drinkers may absorb too much fluoride. Cases have been documented where patients drank 1 to 2 gallons per day of tea for several decades. Non-tea drinkers commonly consume 2-3 mg of fluoride per day from toothpaste, food, and fluoridated water. The official EPA (Environmental Protection Agency, USA) recommendation is to add 0.7 mg of fluoride per liter of water when fluoridating water supplies. This suggests that water fluoridation may be inappropriate or unnecessary for tea drinking populations.

Tannins

Tannins lend an astringent taste and property to tea. Tannins have anti-bacterial properties. As a result, tea is a food treatment for minor bacterial dysentery, gastroenteritis, and dysentery. However, tea may irritate stomach ulcers. Pu-erh has less of a tendency to cause irritation than green tea.

Catechins and Theaflavin

Catechins are naturally occurring phenol antioxidants named after the herb Er Cha (acacia catechu). Catechins are flavanol monomers (a type of flavonoid) and are abundant in both Er Cha and tea. EGCG (epigallocatechin 3-gallate) is a well researched catechin found in tea, especially for its anti-cancer properties. Topical applications of EGCG inhibit cancer growth in UVB induced skin tumors.[52] EGCG has also been shown to inhibit tumor growth when taken internally.[53] EGCG and other monomeric catechins are most abundant in green and white tea because EGCG is converted into thearubigins in the enzymatic oxidation process of making black tea.

Theaflavin, most abundant in black tea, is antioxidative, antiviral, antibacterial and anti-inflammatory.[54] Theaflavin and catechins in green and black tea inhibit HIV. A recent study concludes that, "tea, especially black tea, may be used as a source of anti-HIV agents and theaflavin derivatives may be applied as lead compounds for developing HIV-1 entry inhibitors...."[55] Also,

---

[52] Yao-Ping Lu, You-Rong Lou, Jian-Guo Xie, Qing-Yun Peng, Jie Liao, Chung S. Yang, Mou-Tuan Huang, and Allan H. Conney. Topical applications of caffeine or epigallocatechin gallate (EGCG) inhibit carcinogenesis and selectively increase apoptosis in UVB-induced skin tumors in mice. PNAS. September 17, 2002 vol. 99 no. 19 12455-12460.

[53] Y D Jung, M S Kim, B A Shin, K O Chay, B W Ahn, W Liu, C D Bucana, G E Gallick, and L M Ellis. EGCG, a major component of green tea, inhibits tumour growth by inhibiting VEGF induction in human colon carcinoma cells. Br J Cancer. 2001 March; 84(6): 844–850.

[54] K. Vijayaa, S. Ananthan, and R. Nalini. Antibacterial effect of theaflavin, polyphenon 60 (Camellia sinensis) and Euphorbia hirta on Shigella spp. — a cell culture study. Journal of Ethnopharmacology. Volume 49, Issue 2, 1 December 1995, Pages 115-118.

[55] Shuwen Liua, Hong Lua, Qian Zhaoa, Yuxian Hea, Jinkui Niua, Asim K. Debnatha, Shuguang Wub, , and Shibo Jiang. Theaflavin derivatives in black tea and catechin

theaflavin has been shown to reduce focal cerebral ischemia injuries with its ability to protect neurons from cerebral ischemia.[56]

Tea Facts

- In large population study, tea drinkers were found to have a lower risk of biliary tract cancers and biliary stones.[57]

- A 2001 study published by the American Heart Association concludes that, "Short- and long-term black tea consumption reverses endothelial vasomotor dysfunction in patients with coronary artery disease. This finding may partly explain the association between tea intake and decreased cardiovascular disease events."[58] The study was a joint effort of the Evans Department of Medicine and Whitaker Cardiovascular Institute, Boston University School of Medicine, Boston, Mass, and the Linus Pauling Institute, Oregon State University, Corvallis (B.F.).

- A 1991 study of 9,856 men and 10,233 women found that, "Mean serum cholesterol decreased with increasing tea consumption...." The same study found that the tea drinkers had lower systolic blood pressure. Also, the study found that tea drinkers of one or more cups per day had a slightly lower overall mortality rate. The study was conducted by the National Health Screening Service, Oslo, Norway, the

derivatives in green tea inhibit HIV-1 entry by targeting gp41. Biochimica et Biophysica Acta (BBA) - General Subjects, Volume 1723, Issues 1-3, 25 May 2005, Pages 270-281.
[56] Cai F, Li CR, Wu JL, Chen JG, Liu C, Min Q, Yu W, Ouyang CH, Chen JH. Theaflavin ameliorates cerebral ischemia-reperfusion injury in rats through its anti-inflammatory effect and modulation of STAT-1. Mediators Inflamm. 2006;2006 (5):30490.
[57] Xue-Hong Zhang, Gabriella Andreotti, Yu-Tang Gao, Jie Deng, Enju Liu, Asif Rashid, Kai Wu, Lu Sun, Lori C. Sakoda, Jia-Rong Cheng, Ming-Chang Shen, Bing-Sheng Wang, Tian-Quan Han, Bai-He Zhang, Gloria Gridley, Joseph F. Fraumeni Jr., Ann W. Hsing. Tea drinking and the risk of biliary tract cancers and biliary stones: A population-based case–control study in Shanghai, China. International Journal of Cancer, Volume 118, Issue 12, pages 3089–3094, 15 June 2006.
[58] Stephen J. Duffy, MB, BS, PhD; John F. Keaney Jr, MD; Monika Holbrook, MA; Noyan Gokce, MD; Peter L. Swerdloff, BA; Balz Frei, PhD; Joseph A. Vita, MD. Short- and Long-Term Black Tea Consumption Reverses Endothelial Dysfunction in Patients With Coronary Artery Disease. Circulation. 2001;104:151. Clinical Investigation and Reports. American Heart Association, Inc.

Section for Dietary Research, Institute for Nutrition Research, University of Oslo, Oslo, Norway and the Department of Clinical Chemistry, Ullevål Hospital, Oslo, Norway.[59]

- A study of 61,057 Swedish woman concluded, "that tea consumption is associated with a reduced risk of epithelial ovarian cancer in a dose-response manner." Enrollment for participants was from 1987 to 1990. The participants were screened for cancer through December 2004 with an average follow-up of 15.1 years. Women who seldom or never drank tea were compared with three groups: less than one cup per day, 1 cup per day, 2 or more cups per day. It was concluded that, "tea consumption was inversely associated with the risk of ovarian cancer...." The study also measured that, "Each additional cup of tea per day was associated with an 18% lower risk of ovarian cancer."[60]

- Green tea consumption inhibits lung tumorigenesis and prevents lung tissue DNA lesions due to oxidative damage in mice.[61] 8-hydroxydeoxyguanosine (8-OH-dGuo) is a DNA lesion and green tea prevented its formation in lung tissues. The researchers attributed this phenomenon, at least in part, to green tea's antioxidant properties and EGCG.

- A 2002 study published by the American Heart Association and conducted by researchers at the Beth Israel Deaconess Medical Center, Harvard School of Public Health, and Massachusetts General Hospital concluded that, "tea consumption in tHe Year before acute myocardial infarction is associated with lower mortality after infarction." The study was of 1,900 patients hospitalized with acute myocardial

[59] Inger Stensvold M.Sc., , Aage Tverdal Ph.D., Kari Solvoll B.Sc. and Olav Per Foss M.D. . Tea consumption. Relationship to cholesterol, blood pressure, and coronary and total mortality. Preventive Medicine. Volume 21, Issue 4, July 1992, Pages 546-553.
[60] Susanna C. Larsson, MSc; Alicja Wolk, DMSc. Tea Consumption and Ovarian Cancer Risk in a Population-Based Cohort. Arch Intern Med. 2005;165:2683-2686.
[61] Yong Xu, Chi-Tang Ho, Shantu G. Amin, Chi Han, and Fung-Lung Chung. Inhibition of Tobacco-specific Nitrosamine-induced Lung Tumorigenesis in A/J Mice by Green Tea and Its Major Polyphenol as Antioxidants. Cancer Res July 15, 1992 52; 3875.

infarction between 1989 and 1994. The median follow-up was 3.8 years.[62]

- A 2003 study published in *The American Journal of Cardiology* measured the effects of black tea consumption on coronary flow velocity reserve (CFVR) using transthoracic Doppler echocardiography (TTDE). The study concluded that, "Acute black tea consumption improves coronary vessel function, as determined by CFVR."[63]

- A 1998 study notes that, "a case-control study on breast cancer patients revealed that high daily consumption of green tea was associated with a lower recurrence rate among Stages I and II patients. All the results suggest that consumption of green tea is a practical and effective cancer preventive both before cancer onset and after cancer treatment."[64,65] The study cites EGCG and epicatechin (EC), components of green tea, as having measurable chemotherapeutic effects on lung cancer tissue. The researchers measured that EGCG and EC enhanced apoptosis in lung cancer cells.

- A year 2000 study conducted by the Clinical Gerontology Unit, University of Cambridge School of Medicine, concluded that, "Older women who drank tea had higher BMD (bone mineral density) measurements than did those

[62] Kenneth J. Mukamal, MD, MPH, MA; Malcolm Maclure, ScD; James E. Muller, MD; Jane B. Sherwood, RN; Murray A. Mittleman, MD, DrPH. Tea Consumption and Mortality After Acute Myocardial Infarction. Circulation. 2002;105:2476-2481. doi: 10.1161/01.CIR.0000017201.88994.F7.

[63] Kumiko Hirata, MD, Kenei Shimada, MD, Hiroyuki Watanabe, MD, Ryo Otsuka, MD, Koutaro Tokai, MD, Minoru Yoshiyama, MD, Shunichi Homma, MD, Junichi Yoshikawa, MD. Black tea increases coronary flow velocity reserve in healthy male subjects. American Journal of Cardiology. Volume 93, Issue 11 , Pages 1384-1388, 1 June 2004.

[64] Masami Suganuma, Sachiko Okabe, Naoko Sueoka, Eisaburo Sueoka, Satoru Matsuyama, Kazue Imai, Kei Nakachi and Hirota Fujiki. Green tea and cancer chemoprevention. Mutation Research/Fundamental and Molecular Mechanisms of Mutagenesis. Volume 428, Issues 1-2, 16 July 1999, Pages 339-344.

[65] Dugald Seely, ND, MSc Cand. The Effects of Green Tea Consumption on Incidence of Breast Cancer and Recurrence of Breast Cancer: A Systematic Review and Meta-analysis. Integr Cancer Ther. June 2005 vol. 4 no. 2 144-155.

who did not drink tea. Nutrients found in tea, such as flavonoids, may influence BMD. Tea drinking may protect against osteoporosis in older women." The study was conducted with a patient sample size of 1,256 women between the ages of 65-76 years of age. Bone mineral density was higher in the areas measured in the study: lumbar spine, femoral neck, greater trochanter, Ward's triangle.[66] Ward's triangle is the bone of the femoral head region.

Tea Nutrients

Black Tea, brewed, prepared with distilled water		
Source: USDA National Nutrient Database for Standard Reference		
Nutrient	Units	Value per 100 grams
Minerals		
Iron, Fe	mg	0.01
Magnesium, Mg	mg	1
Phosphorus, P	mg	1
Potassium, K	mg	21
Sodium, Na	mg	0
Zinc, Zn	mg	0.01
Copper, Cu	mg	0.008
Manganese, Mn	mg	0.219
Vitamins		
Riboflavin	mg	0.014
Pantothenic acid	mg	0.011
Folate, total	mcg	5
Folate, food	mcg	5
Folate, DFE	mcg_DFE	5
Other		
Caffeine	mg	20

Common Contraindications

- Tea stimulates the central nervous system and clears the Shen. However, it is not recommended after dinner as it may cause insomnia due to its caffeine content.

---

[66] Verona M Hegarty, Helen M May and Kay-Tee Khaw. Tea drinking and bone mineral density in older women. American Journal of Clinical Nutrition, Vol. 71, No. 4, 1003-1007, April 2000.

- Tea consumption interferes with iron absorption. It is generally not recommended for iron deficient patients or children.

- Caffeinated products may aggravate the lining of the stomach or duodenum and promote the secretion of acid. Tea is not recommended for patients with a stomach ulcer or duodenal ulcer.

- Tea is consumed when freshly made and loses medicinal benefits when stored overnight. Canned and bottled tea products are an exception to the rule in that they are sealed.

- Water, not tea, is appropriate for assisting in the consumption of pharmaceutical drugs. Tea has many chemical ingredients and may interfere with absorption.

- Tea consumption by breast-feeding mothers may interfere with lactation and may lead to overstimulation of the baby. It is recommended to curb or halt tea consumption.

- Patients with irregular heartbeats are recommended to avoid drinking tea. Tea may worsen the condition.

Tea Combinations and Applications

Pu-erh Tea with Fang Feng
Pu-erh   9-12 grams.
Fang Feng   9-12 grams.
Boil the combination for 1-2 minutes. This is effective for treating Tou Feng (Head Wind) headaches. Tou Feng headaches are caused by exposure to external wind. Like the wind, the pain moves to different locations. This home remedy is also useful for the treatment of headaches due to allergies.

Green Tea with Mint, Lemon, or Honey
Green tea prepared with mint, lemon, and/or honey is often used to soothe a parched or sore throat.

Green Tea External Soak

Green tea may be applied to external infections, eczema with discharge, and poison oak. Soak a towel in cold green tea and wash the affected area with the tea. This home remedy helps the burning to subside and reduces discharge.

Geng Mi Cha (Geng Mai Cha, Brown Rice Tea)

Geng Mi Cha is green tea with dry-fried rice. The rice is prepared with the chao method, stir-frying the rice without liquid. Geng Mi Cha becomes less cooling as a result of the frying process. In some preparations of Geng Mi Cha, the temperature becomes neutral or warming. The fried rice's warming effects often protect the Stomach Qi from digestive irritation associated with green tea consumption. The fried rice has a mild tonify Spleen Qi function. Historically, millet was dry-fried and added to green tea. Corn and other grains can also be used. Geng Mi Cha is popular in Japan.

Green Tea with Citrus Peel for Hangovers

Combine green tea with Ju Hong or Chen Pi for the treatment of headache, nausea, and malaise due to prior excess alcohol consumption. Add the ingredients to the cup, add hot water, and drink.

Simplified Chuan Xiong Cha Tiao San

Combine 1.5-3g of Chuan Xiong with green tea. Place the ingredients in a cup, add hot water, and drink. This is for the treatment of minor cases of wind attack including wind-cold headaches and sinus congestion. Best results are achieved when taken at least one hour after meals because the wind-attack affects the upper jiao (burner). Green tea is also consumed when taking the patent formula Chuan Xiong Cha Tiao San.

Shi Ye Cha (Persimmon Leaf Tea)

Persimmon leaf with hot water is a traditional beverage. Historically, collecting the leaves from nearby trees was considered an alternative to purchasing tea. Village farmers drinking this tea often did not suffer from high blood pressure. Research shows that persimmon leaf (Shi Ye) has hypolipidemic effects.[67] To enhance the flavor, mix tea with persimmon leaves.

Research shows that oral consumption of persimmon leaf extract effectively reduces the presentation of atopic dermatitis, inhibits histamine release, and reduces serum IgE levels.[68]

Longjing Ju Hua Cha

Mix Longjing green tea or another variety of green tea with Ju Hua (Chrysanthemum), Shan Zha (Hawthorne Fruit) and Chen Pi (Tangerine Peel). This is a food treatment for high blood pressure and high cholesterol levels. Longjing Cha (Dragon Well Tea) is a variety of green tea from Hangzhou, Zhejiang Province, China. Also, a traditional shrimp dish is prepared with Longjing tea leaves. It is a local delicacy of Hangzhou.

Xiao Ku Cao Jue Ming Cha

Mix Xia Ku Cao and Jue Ming Zi with any variety of tea. Xia Ku Cao has a mild flavor and can be added whole or chopped. Jue Ming Zi requires grinding because it is a firm seed. This tea is appropriate as a dietary supplement for those with high blood pressure due to Liver Fire. Note: Jue Ming Zi is often consumed without other herbs or tea as a weight loss tea and for relieving constipation. Alternately, Chao Jue Ming Zi is a dry-roasted preparation of the herb that can be added to tea. Dry-roasted Jue Ming Zi provides a nice flavor and aroma.

---

[67] J.S. Leea, M.K. Leeb, T.Y. Hac, S.H. Bokd, H.M. Parke, K.S. Jeongf, M.N. Woog, G.-M. Dog, J.-Y. Yeog and M.-S. Choig. Supplementation of whole persimmon leaf improves lipid profiles and suppresses body weight gain in rats fed high-fat diet. Food and Chemical Toxicology. Volume 44, Issue 11, November 2006, Pages 1875-1883.

[68] Mayumi Kotani, BSc, Motonobu Matsumoto, BSc, Akihito Fujita, BSc, Shinji Higa, MD, Way Wang, MD, PhD, Masaki Suemura, MD, PhD, Tadamitsu Kishimoto, MD, PhD, Toshio Tanaka, MD, PhD. Persimmon leaf extract and astragalin inhibit development of dermatitis and IgE elevation in NC/Nga mice. The Journal of Allergy and Clinical Immunology. Volume 106, Issue 1, Pages 159-166, July 2000.

Jiang Cha Wu Mei Yin

Combine 2-3 slices Sheng Jiang (fresh ginger), 2-3 pieces of Wu Mei (sour plum), and green tea. This preparation is a home remedy for the treatment of chronic coughs and loose stools. Wu Mei is astringent and helps to consolidate Lung Qi to relieving coughing and to treat diarrhea.

Another popular home remedy for the treatment of chronic coughs combines He Zi, Pang Da Hai, and green tea. This is also used for the treatment of a chronic sore throat and laryngitis. To use, put the ingredients in a cup and add hot water. The Pang Da Hai will expand and the flesh of the fruit can be eaten. Pang Da Hai treats hoarseness of the voice due to Lung Heat, hot phlegm, or Lung Yin deficiency. He Zi is astringent and also treats hoarseness of the voice. This mild combination can be used regularly and is particularly useful to those who speak or sing often.

Zhu Ye Mai Dong Cha

Combine dry or fresh bamboo leaves with Mai Men Dong and green tea. This tea can be consumed daily for the treatment of Yin deficiency and it promotes the production of bodily fluids (Jin Ye). It is useful for the treatment of menopausal and diabetic syndromes.

Shan Zha Hong Cha

Combine a healthy amount of Shan Zha (hawthorn berry) with any variety of tea. Steep, then add Hong Tang (red sugar, crystallized cane juice). This sweet and sour tea is available as a pre-package product in Asian markets. However, many brands use an excessive quantity of sugar. Shan Zha removes food stagnation and this tea is helpful for children who have overeaten. Clinical grade Sha Zha usually contains seeds, however, dietetics grade Shan Zha (often found in Asian markets) has been cleaned and does not contain seeds. Use the seedless variety. Modern research shows that Shan Zha is helpful in reducing triglyceride and cholesterol levels.[69]

Lou Bo Cha

Combine sliced daikon (Lou Bou) with tea to make a soup or cup of tea. Drink the liquid and eat the daikon. Similar to Lai Fu Zi (radish seed), daikon radish removes food stagnation and descends the Qi.

Lian Zi Xin Cha

Combine Lian Zi Xin with green tea and steep. This is a food treatment for Heart Fire and Heart and Kidney not communicating. Lian Zi Xin is the heart of the lotus seed and is a *heart to heart* treatment according to Chinese medicine principles.

---

[69] Hong X, Hou-En Xu, Damien Ryan. A Study of the Comparative Effects of Hawthorn Fruit Compound and Simvastatin on Lowering Blood Lipid Levels. Volume: 37, Issue: 5(2009) pp. 903-908.

Fungi

Bai Mu Er and Hei Mu Er

Bai Mu Er (Yin Er, White Wood Ear, Fructificatio Tremellae Fuciformis, White Fungus) is sweet, bland and neutral. Bai Mu Er enters the Lung and Stomach channels and nourishes Lung Qi and Yin. Hei Mu Er (Black Fungus, Auricularia Polytricha, Black Wood Ear Fungus) is sweet, bland, neutral and enters the Stomach and Large Intestine channels. Hei Mu Er nourishes and invigorates blood and nourishes Lung Qi and Yin. Both fungi tonify Qi, nourish Yin, and generate fluids. Bai Mu Er more strongly nourishes Lung Qi and Yin whereas Hei Mu Er nourishes and invigorates blood. Bai Mu Er and Hei Mu Er are prepared in sweet dessert soups made with rock sugar. They are also common in savory entrees including stews, soups, and stir-fries.

Hei Mu Er has been shown to reduce cholesterol and triglycerides including significant reductions of LDL cholesterol.[70] Hei Mu Er inhibits platelet aggregation and thins the blood.[71] Another study notes that, "Administration of black fungus polysaccharides had significantly enhanced myocardium and blood antioxidant enzyme activities and reduced lipid peroxidation level in high fat mice. Our results indicated that black fungus polysaccharides could be beneficial for protection against cardiovascular diseases and its complications."[72] Hei Mu Er has also been shown to have anti-tumor properties.[73]

---

[70] Byung-Keun Yang, Ji-Young Ha, Sang-Chul Jeong, Young-Jae Jeon, Kyung-Soo Ra, Surajit Das, Jong-Won Yun and Chi-Hyun Song. Hypolipidemic effect of an exo-biopolymer produced from submerged mycelial culture of Auricularia polytricha in rats. BIOTECHNOLOGY LETTERS. Volume 24, Number 16, 1319-1325.

[71] Hokama Y, Hokama JL. In vitro inhibition of platelet aggregation with low dalton compounds from aqueous dialysates of edible fungi. Res Commun Chem Pathol Pharmacol. 1981 Jan;31(1):177-80.

[72] Ma Jiangweia, Qiao Zengyong, and Xiang Xia. Optimization of extraction procedure for black fungus polysaccharides and effect of the polysaccharides on blood lipid and myocardium antioxidant enzymes activities. Carbohydrate Polymers. Volume 84, Issue 3, 17 March 2011, Pages 1061-1068.

[73] Mengyao Yu, Xiaoyan Xu, Yuan Qing, Xia Luo, Zhirong Yang and Linyong Zheng. Isolation of an anti-tumor polysaccharide from Auricularia polytricha (jew's ear) and its

Ling Zhi

Ling Zhi (Ganoderma Japonicum) is a mushroom that is sweet, neutral and enters the Lung, Heart, Liver and Spleen channels. Ling Zhi tonifies the Qi and Blood, benefits the Spleen and Stomach, calms the spirit (Shen), benefits the brain and intelligence; tonifies Lung Qi and stops coughing and wheezing. Generally, this mushroom is boiled in water to extract the ingredients but is not eaten. However, some powdered preparations call for eating the powder.

There are five major varieties of Ling Zhi and over 150 varieties in totality. Red and brown Ling Zhi are common. Another variety has a shiny black surface. Ling Zhi may also be blue-green, red, yellow, white, or purple. Ling Zhi is translated as spiritual mushroom and gets its name in part due to its ability to treat illness and save lives. Ling means both powerful and spiritual. One variety, known as turkey tail (trametes versicolor), grows on large trees. A normal dose is approximately 3 to 15 grams per day.

- Ling Zhi is helpful for treating immunity disorders characterized by chronic infections with low white blood cell counts. Ling Zhi increases the white cell blood count.

- Ling Zhi treats heart disorders with blood stagnation and/or chest bi pain. Ling Zhi treats a variety of cardiovascular disorders due to deficiency, strengthens the heart and improves cardiac function.

- Ling Zhi treats high blood pressure and lowers cholesterol and triglyceride levels.

- Ling Zhi adjusts the blood pressure to regulate the heartbeat.

- Ling Zhi treats dyslipidemia with deficiency of Qi and Blood.

- Ling Zhi has antineoplastic properties.

effects on macrophage activation. EUROPEAN FOOD RESEARCH AND TECHNOLOGY. Volume 228, Number 3, 477-485.

- Ling Zhi is useful in the treatment of chronic asthma and for the treatment of chronic coughing with phlegm or due to Yin deficiency dryness.

Shiitake Mushroom (Xianggu, Donggu, Huagu)

Shiitake mushrooms are tasty and are sold both in fresh and dried preparations. They are native to East Asia, very popular throughout Japan, and are now primarily produced in China. Shiitake has a similar but slightly weaker function than Ling Zhi in its ability to benefit the immune system and to lower cholesterol. Shiitake is a great source of iron, B3, B5, B6, B2, manganese, phosphorus, fiber, and potassium in the diet. Laboratory studies suggest that Shitake mushrooms, like many edible mushrooms, have anti-cancer benefits.

Monkey Head Mushroom (Hou Tou Bu, Bear Head Mushroom)

Like many varieties of edible mushrooms, the Monkey Head mushroom lowers blood lipid levels and benefits the immune system. Hou is translated as monkey, tou is head and gu is mushroom.

Fruits, Vegetables, Herbs

Gou Qi Ye

Gou Qi Ye (lycium leaf) has similar properties as Gou Qi Zi (lycium fruit). Use the leaf as a vegetable. It is often boiled in soups with a little salt and oil added.

Gou Qi Zi tonifies the blood and benefits the eyes. Gou Qi Zi is traditionally added to desserts.

Zi Su Ye

Zi Su Ye (perilla leaf) is traditionally served with sushi to prevent seafood poisoning, allergic reactions, rashes, nausea, vomiting, and itching. It may also be combined with tea as a beverage. In sushi restaurants, it is often substituted with a plastic leaf used for ornamental purposes.

Xi Yang Shen (Hua Qi Shen, American Ginseng)

Xi Yang Shen often made into a beverage to nourish Qi, Yin, and promote body fluids. Its cooling nature distinguishes itself from Ren Shen (Radix Ginseng). Xi Yang Shen has less of a tonify Qi function and consequently has less side effects.

Xi Yang Cai (Watercress)

Xi Yang Cai is cold, nourishes the Lungs, alleviates constipation and is valued for its significant nutritional and medicinal benefits. Xi Yang Cai is in the cabbage family and is a popular garnish in the USA. It is often served blanched or in soups throughout China. It is also cut and lightly sprinkled on salads. Xi Yang Cai is served freshly juiced with a little salt added. The juice is a helpful home remedy for the treatment of dry coughs or coughing with blood. Cooking Xi Yang Cai in oil diminishes its medicinal functions. Xi Yang Chai combines well with dry or fresh figs, Mi Zao (honey date), Gou Qi Zi (lycium berry), and Chen Pi (aged citrus peel). It is spicy in its raw form but is mild and sweet when cooked. Watercress contains PEITC-NAC (N-acetylcysteine conjugate of phenethyl isothiocyanate) that has been shown to inhibit the proliferation of prostate cancer and tumorigenesis.[74]

Watercress, raw				
Source: USDA National Nutrient Database for Standard Reference				
Nutrient	Units	Value per 100 grams	1 cup, chopped ------- 34g	10 sprigs ------- 25g
Energy	kcal	11	4	3
Energy	kJ	46	16	12
Protein	g	2.30	0.78	0.57
Total lipid (fat)	g	0.10	0.03	0.03
Ash	g	1.20	0.41	0.30
Carbohydrate, by difference	g	1.29	0.44	0.32
Fiber, total dietary	g	0.5	0.2	0.1
Sugars, total	g	0.20	0.07	0.05
Minerals				
Calcium, Ca	mg	120	41	30
Iron, Fe	mg	0.20	0.07	0.05
Magnesium, Mg	mg	21	7	5
Phosphorus, P	mg	60	20	15
Potassium, K	mg	330	112	82
Sodium, Na	mg	41	14	10
Zinc, Zn	mg	0.11	0.04	0.03
Copper, Cu	mg	0.077	0.026	0.019
Manganese, Mn	mg	0.244	0.083	0.061
Selenium, Se	mcg	0.9	0.3	0.2
Vitamins				
Vitamin C, total ascorbic acid	mg	43.0	14.6	10.8
Thiamin	mg	0.090	0.031	0.022
Riboflavin	mg	0.120	0.041	0.030
Niacin	mg	0.200	0.068	0.050
Pantothenic acid	mg	0.310	0.105	0.077
Vitamin B-6	mg	0.129	0.044	0.032
Folate, total	mcg	9	3	2
Folate, food	mcg	9	3	2
Folate, DFE	mcg_DFE	9	3	2

[74] Jen Wei Chiao, Hongyan Wu, Gita Ramaswamy, C. Clifford Conaway, Fung-Lung Chung, Longgui Wang and Delong Liu. Ingestion of an isothiocyanate metabolite from cruciferous vegetables inhibits growth of human prostate cancer cell xenografts by apoptosis and cell cycle arrest. Oxford Journals, Life Sciences & Medicine, Carcinogenesis Volume 25, Issue 8 p. 1403-1408.

Choline, total	mg	9.0	3.1	2.2
Vitamin A, RAE	mcg_RAE	160	54	40
Retinol	mcg	0	0	0
Carotene, beta	mcg	1914	651	478
Vitamin A, IU	IU	3191	1085	798
Lutein + zeaxanthin	mcg	5767	1961	1442
Vitamin E (alpha-tocopherol)	mg	1.00	0.34	0.25
Vitamin K (phylloquinone)	mcg	250.0	85.0	62.5
Lipids				
Fatty acids, total saturated	g	0.027	0.009	0.007
Fatty acids, total monounsaturated	g	0.008	0.003	0.002
Fatty acids, total polyunsaturated	g	0.035	0.012	0.009
Cholesterol	mg	0	0	0
Amino acids				
Tryptophan	g	0.030	0.010	0.007
Threonine	g	0.133	0.045	0.033
Isoleucine	g	0.093	0.032	0.023
Leucine	g	0.166	0.056	0.042
Lysine	g	0.134	0.046	0.034
Methionine	g	0.020	0.007	0.005
Cystine	g	0.007	0.002	0.002
Phenylalanine	g	0.114	0.039	0.029
Tyrosine	g	0.063	0.021	0.016
Valine	g	0.137	0.047	0.034
Arginine	g	0.150	0.051	0.037
Histidine	g	0.040	0.014	0.010
Alanine	g	0.137	0.047	0.034
Aspartic acid	g	0.187	0.064	0.047
Glutamic acid	g	0.190	0.065	0.048
Glycine	g	0.112	0.038	0.028
Proline	g	0.096	0.033	0.024
Serine	g	0.060	0.020	0.015

Bok Choy

Bok Choy is in the cabbage family and includes varieties such as baby bok choy and napa cabbage. It has similar functions as watercress but is less cooling. It is slightly cool to neutral. Fresh bok choy is often stir-fried or put in soups. Modern research shows that bok choy has antioxidant and anti-cancer properties.[75] Bok

---

[75] Sang-Ah Lee, Jay H Fowke, Wei Lu, Chuangzhong Ye, Ying Zheng, Qiuyin Cai, Kai Gu, Yu-Tang Gao, Xiao-ou Shu and Wei Zheng.Cruciferous vegetables, the GSTP1

Choy is an excellent source of absorbable calcium.[76] Bok choy is one of the most commonly consumed vegetables in China and is a staple vegetable in the Korean side-dish kimchi.

Tong Cai (Ipomoea aquatica, Convolvulaceae; Tong Choy, Ong Tung Tsoi, Water Spinach, Chinese Spinach)

This green vegetable is very popular in Southeast Asia. It is very cooling and gently promotes bowel movements. Its cooling nature makes this food well suited for diabetics with deficiency heat symptoms. For medicinal purposes, the plant can be boiled and the resultant liquid can be consumed without the need to eat the vegetable. Tong Cai is very cooling and excess consumption of the liquid may cause deficiency. If the patient feels tired or dizzy after consumption, add 3-6 grams of Korean or American ginseng powder to the liquid to prevent side effects.

This plant is a healthy addition to egg drop soup and many other soups. Tong Cai is often boiled, steamed, stir-fried or pickled. Tong Cai combines well with onions, chilies, garlic, shrimp paste, ginger, and oyster sauce. Possession of Tong Cai is prohibited in Florida because overgrowth has blocked aqueducts, lakes, and other waterways.

Vietnamese Spinach (Malabar Spinach, Red Vine Spinach, Basella Alba, Mong Toi)

Vietnamese spinach is cooling and gently promotes bowel movements. A quality source of fiber, it is rich in vitamins A and C, iron and calcium. It is commonly added to soups and stir-fries. Vietnamese spinach combines well with tofu, seafood, garlic and chili peppers. Vietnamese spinach has a mucilaginous property that acts as a thickener for soups.

Ile105Val genetic polymorphism, and breast cancer risk. American Journal of Clinical Nutrition, Vol. 87, No. 3, 753-760, March 2008.

[76] R.P. HEANEY, C.M. WEAVER, SM. HINDERS, B. MARTIN, P.T. PACKARD. Absorbability of Calcium from Brassica Vegetables: Broccoli, Bok Choy, and Kale. Journal of Food Science. Volume 58, Issue 6, pages 1378–1380, November 1993.

Ku Gua (Bitter Melon, Bitter Gourd, Balsam-Pear)

This fruit grows throughout Asia. Ku Gua is extremely bitter. Its temperature is very cold. In Asia, it is juiced in the summertime for its cooling effects with watermelon, honey or cucumber. Ku Gua clears heat toxins similarly to the function of Pu Gong Ying (dandelion). Ku Gua is added to soups and is often cooked with meats.

- Drinking Ku Gua juice straight or combined with cucumber is recommended for the treatment of skin infections and acne.

- Ku Gua helps to preserve the smoothness of skin and prevents roughness.

- Juiced or eaten, Ku Gua assists in losing excess weight. A 'tea' is made from Ku Gua that is helpful for weight loss.

- According to Chinese medicine principles, diabetes is associated with pathological sweetness and the bitter flavor beneficially balances diabetics. Ku Gua is indicated for diabetics.

- Ku Gua has anti-HIV and anti-tumor functions. Researchers from the Department of Biochemistry (New York University School of Medicine), American BioSciences, National Institute of Child Health and Human Development, and the Laboratory of Biochemical Physiology (Biological Response Modifiers Program, DCT, National Cancer Institute-Frederick Cancer Research and Development Center) note that "MAP30 is an anti-HIV plant protein that we have identified and purified to homogeneity from bitter melon (Momordica charantia). It is capable of acting against multiple stages of the viral life cycle, on acute infection as well as replication in chronically infected cells. In addition to antiviral action, MAP30 also possesses anti-tumor activity, topological inactivation of viral DNA, inhibition of viral integrase and cell-free ribosome-inactivation activities." [77]

Balsam-pear (bitter gourd), pods, cooked, boiled, drained, without salt			
Source: USDA National Nutrient Database for Standard Reference			
Nutrient	**Units**	**Value per 100 grams**	**0.5 cup ------- 62g**
Minerals			
Calcium, Ca	mg	9	6
Iron, Fe	mg	0.38	0.24
Magnesium, Mg	mg	16	10
Phosphorus, P	mg	36	22
Potassium, K	mg	319	198
Sodium, Na	mg	6	4
Zinc, Zn	mg	0.77	0.48
Copper, Cu	mg	0.033	0.020
Manganese, Mn	mg	0.086	0.053
Selenium, Se	mcg	0.2	0.1
Vitamins			
Vitamin C, total ascorbic acid	mg	33.0	20.5
Thiamin	mg	0.051	0.032
Riboflavin	mg	0.053	0.033
Niacin	mg	0.280	0.174
Pantothenic acid	mg	0.193	0.120
Vitamin B-6	mg	0.041	0.025
Folate, total	mcg	51	32
Folate, food	mcg	51	32
Folate, DFE	mcg_DFE	51	32
Choline, total	mg	10.8	6.7
Vitamin A, RAE	mcg_RAE	6	4
Carotene, beta	mcg	68	42
Vitamin A, IU	IU	113	70
Lutein + zeaxanthin	mcg	1323	820
Vitamin E (alpha-tocopherol)	mg	0.14	0.09
Vitamin K (phylloquinone)	mcg	4.8	3.0

---

[77] Sylvia Lee-Huanga, , Paul L. Huangb, Hao-Chia Chenc, Philip L. Huangb, Aldar Bourinbaiara, Henry I. Huang and Hsiang-fu Kung. Anti-HIV and anti-tumor activities of recombinant MAP30 from bitter melon. Gene. Volume 161, Issue 2, 19 August 1995, Pages 151-156.

Dong Gua (Winter Melon, Wax Gourd)

Winter Melon has properties and functions similar to that of Fu Ling. It is sweet, bland and cooling. Dong Gua promotes urination, drains dampness, treats edema and is excellent for cooling in the summertime. Winter Melon is native to Southeast Asia and has a long shelf life due in part to its waxy coating. Winter Melon has an external appearance similar to that of a watermelon and it has white flesh.

- Dong Gua Zhong: Cut the Dong Gua in half lengthwise. Remove the seeds from the core and add dried scallops, chicken, and mushrooms to the center of one half. Double boil or steam the Dong Gua with the ingredients. The flesh becomes very soft when cooked. Serve and enjoy!

- Make a soup by adding Yi Yi Ren and Chen Pi. Shan Yao can also be added. This soup promotes urination and drains dampness.

- The Winter Melon seed (Dong Gua Ren, Dong Gua Zi, Wax Gourd Seed) is used in Chinese medicine herbal decoctions for the treatment of lung and intestinal abscesses due to damp-heat with phlegm. Winter melon seed is also used to treat damp-heat leukorrhea.

Xi Gua (Watermelon)

Xi Gua is sweet and cold. It enters the Heart, Stomach, and Urination Bladder channels. Xi Gua clears summer heat and dampness, quenches thirst, and promotes urination. The fruit may be eaten when ripe or may be pickled.

- Unripened watermelon has a stronger function and may be used to reduce high blood pressure. Slice the watermelon and boil the red flesh in water with the rind and add vinegar to increase the function. The white part of the rind is particularly useful in the treatment of high blood pressure.

- A 2011 study published in the *American Journal of Hypertension* demonstrates "that watermelon supplementation improves aortic hemodynamics....″[78] This study was comprised of researchers from the Department of Nutrition, Food and Exercise Sciences, College of Human Sciences, Florida State University; and the Department of Horticultural Sciences, College of Agriculture and Life Sciences, North Carolina State University.

Cucumbers

Huang Gua (Yellow Melon) and Qing Gua (Greenish Yellow Melon)

Ripe cucumbers are green. Cucumbers turn yellow if left on the vine. The older yellow cucumbers are tougher and have a stronger medicinal function. Cucumbers are cool, sweet and enter the Lung, Stomach and Large Intestine channels. Cucumbers clear Lung and Stomach heat. For a stronger medicinal effect, boil yellow cucumbers with cooling herbs to make a soup. Cucumber juice may be applied externally to soothe heat related skin conditions.

Pu Gong Ying (Dandelion)

Pu Gong Ying is bitter, sweet and cold and enters the Liver and Stomach channels. Pu Gong Ying clears heat and toxins. Dandelion clears skin disorders and abscesses. Dietetics use of Pu Gong Ying is particularly beneficial for treating Gallbladder related issues including gallstones and damp-heat jaundice.

Use the entire plant including the root. Wash the plant and cut it into small pieces. Boil with a little olive oil and add salt. Eat the plant and drink the soup. The western style of using dandelion greens in salads has a weak medicinal function.

Ma Chi Xian (Purslane)

Ma Chi Xian is sour, cold and enters the Large Intestine and Liver channels. Ma Chi Xian clears heat and toxins and cools the Blood.

---

[78] Arturo Figueroa, Marcos A. Sanchez-Gonzalez, Penelope M. Perkins-Veazie and Bahram H. Arjmandi. Effects of Watermelon Supplementation on Aortic Blood Pressure and Wave Reflection in Individuals With Prehypertension: A Pilot Study. American Journal of Hypertension 2011; 24 1, 40–44.

Ma Chi Xian treats damp-heat in the Large Intestine including diarrhea conditions such as dysentery. Ma Chi Xian treats blood Lin syndrome (blood in the urine). For patients with damp and cold in the Stomach and Spleen, Ma Chi Xian may cause loose stool. Ma Chi Xian is used in salads. For a stronger medicinal effect, boil the whole plant in a small amount of water. A small amount of water is used so that the entire soup can be consumed. Eat the plant and drink the soup. Modern research shows that Purslane has detoxifying properties from bisphenol A exposure.

Jie Cai (Mustard Greens, Brassica Juncea)

Jie Cai is spicy, warming and has a distinctly pungent odor. Jie Cai enters the Lung and Stomach channels. Similar to Bai Jie Zi (white mustard seed), Jie Cai is useful for the treatment of coughs due to wind-cold.

- • For the treatment of beginning stage wind-cold coughs: Boil a hard boiled egg with some sliced beef. Next, add two slices of Sheng Jiang (fresh ginger) and then add Jie Cai. Eat the mustard greens and drink the soup.

Jiu Cai (Chinese Chives, Garlic Chives, Allium Tuberosum)

Chinese Chives are stems and leaves that are similar in appearance to green onions and have a flavor similar to that of garlic. Jiu Cai has an invigorate blood function when consumed raw and has a tonify Yang function, similar to that of Jiu Cai Zi (Chinese Chive seed), when cooked. Jiu Cai is spicy, warm and enters the Liver, Stomach, and Kidney channels. Jiu Cai is usually chopped into small pieces and cooked. It is common in stews, soups, stir-fries. Jiu Cai combines well with eggs and seafood.

- • For impotence, infertility, and sexual function disorder due to Kidney Yang deficiency: Combine chopped Jiu Cai with shrimp and scrambled egg. First scramble the eggs, then add the Chinese Chives and prepared shrimp. This egg foo young method is a type of Chinese Chive omelet. Eggs are related to Jing and shrimp tonifies Yang and Jing. Chinese medicine theory notes that shrimp lay many eggs making them related to Jing.

- Chinese Chive fiber supplement to treat constipation: Boil uncut Chinese Chives until soft and remove from the water. Eat the Chinese Chives and add soy sauce for flavor. There is an old story about a child who ate a pocketknife that opened when ingested. The child was instructed to eat Chinese Chives. The Chinese Chives wrapped around the knife, closed it, and the knife was eliminated in the stool while wrapped in the Chinese Chives. To this day, Chinese Chives are often chopped because the fiber is eliminated in the stool.

- To invigorate the blood for the treatment of minor injuries or to relieve Chest Bi Pain due to coronary arteriole sclerosis: Juice a bunch of raw chives in a juicing machine and drink. The blood invigorating function helps to relieve pain.

Ge Gen (Kudzu Root)

Ge Gen is native to Southeast Asia and Japan. It grows in the Southeastern US and preserves the same medicinal functions. Ge Gen is sweet, cool, pungent and enters the Spleen and Stomach channels. Ge Gen expels wind, releases the muscles, clears heat, generates fluids (Jin Ye), stops diarrhea, and promotes the release of pathogens through eruptions (especially for the treatment of measles).

- To promote Jin Ye (fluids): Make a soup with fresh Ge Gen. Eat the Ge Gen and drink the soup.

- To nourish Yin: Chop fresh Ge Gen into pieces and add dried seafood (conch, oyster…), meat (lean pork, chicken…) and make a soup.

Lotus Root (Ou Jie, Lotus Rhizome)

Ou Jie is sweet and astringent. Cooking Ou Jie lends a slightly warm property to the herb, fresh Ou Jie is cooling and the dried herb is neutral. Fresh Ou Jie is more astringent than the dried herb.

Ou Jie enters the Lung, Stomach, and Liver channels. Ou Jie stops bleeding. Ou Jie is common in soups and sautés.

- For coughing with blood or any bleeding disorder: The astringent properties of fresh lotus root juice make it suitable for the treatment of bleeding disorders.

- For the treatment of bleeding disorders and bleeding related to the stomach and ulcerative colitis: Cut the lotus root into small pieces, add cuttlefish and make a soup. Optional ingredients include adzuki beans (Chi Xiao Dou), mung beans (Lu Dou), and green beans.

Celery

Chinese celery has a smaller stem than western celery. Both have the same medicinal properties. Celery is bitter, sweet, pungent and cooling. Celery enters the Liver and Stomach channels and pacifies Liver heat. Celery may also be used to treat Liver Yin deficiency with Yang uprising including symptoms such as redness of the face and irritability. Celery has its strongest medicinal function when consumed raw. Celery may be juiced, added to salads, boiled, and stir-fried. Celery is used in Chinese medicine dietetics to lower blood pressure and modern research demonstrates that celery reduces total serum cholesterol.[79]

Daikon Radish (Qing Luo Bo)

The daikon radish typically has either a white flesh or green flesh. Qing (green) Bo is more bitter than the white variety. Daikon is spicy, sweet, cooling and enters the Lung and Stomach channels. Luo Bo benefits digestion and dissolves phlegm.

- Fresh daikon juice (Luo Bo Zhi) benefits the Lungs to treat coughing, coughing with phlegm and other respiratory ailments. Lemon juice, mint, and honey can be added to enhance the medicinal benefits and to adjust the flavor.

---

[79] Tsi D, Tan BK. The mechanism underlying the hypocholesterolaemic activity of aqueous celery extract, its butanol and aqueous fractions in genetically hypercholesterolaemic RICO rats. Life Sci. 2000 Jan 14;66(8):755-67.

- Fresh daikon juice with celery is a food treatment for high blood pressure.

- Cooked daikon radish, similar in function to daikon seeds (Lai Fu Zi, Luo Bo Zi), treats food stagnation and is beneficial for digestion disorders. The fiber content invigorates a sluggish stomach. Daikon is commonly prepared with tofu.

- White Tiger Soup or Green Dragon White Tiger Soup treats coughing, prevents the common cold & 'flu' and is particularly beneficial in the summertime to benefit the skin and for the treatment of acne. Make a soup with daikon and fresh green olives. Fresh olives can be substituted with He Zi or mung beans (Lu Dou) when they are not available. Mung beans are particularly beneficial for the treatment of skin conditions.

- Daikon radish is often pickled in Japanese cuisine.

Carrot (Red Carrot, Hong Luo Bo)

According to five elements principles, the red-yellow (orange) color combination reflects that carrots enter the Heart and Spleen channels. Carrots are sweet, neutral, tonify the Qi and Blood of the entire body, and benefit the Ying Qi (nutrition Qi). Carrots benefit vision and treat night blindness.

Carrots have a similar shape and function to that of ginseng and are nicknamed "poor people ginseng." Carrots are rich in beta-carotene (a vitamin A precursor) and other carotenoids, vitamin C, B vitamins, iron, magnesium, phosphorus, calcium and potassium. Excess consumption of carrots may lead to carotenosis. Although benign and reversible, the skin turns orange for the duration of the illness.

- To tonify Qi and Blood, slice carrots and make a soup. Drink the soup and eat the carrots. Cooking makes the carrots easier to absorb.

- In the west, carrots are often juiced.

- Carrots reduce cholesterol and triglycerides. A 1997 study published in the American Journal of Clinical Nutrition notes, "Two hundred grams of raw carrot eaten at breakfast each day for 3 weeks significantly reduced serum cholesterol by 11%, increased fecal bile acid and fat excretion by 50%, and modestly increased stool weight by 25%. This suggests an associated change in bacterial flora or metabolism. The changes in serum cholesterol, fecal bile acids, and fat persisted 3 weeks after stopping treatment."[80]

Carrots			
Source: USDA National Nutrient Database for Standard Reference			
Nutrient	**Units**	**Cooked, Boiled, Drained** Value per 100g	**Raw** Value per 100g
Minerals			
Calcium, Ca	mg	30	33
Iron, Fe	mg	0.34	0.30
Magnesium, Mg	mg	10	12
Phosphorus, P	mg	30	35
Potassium, K	mg	235	320
Sodium, Na	mg	58	69
Zinc, Zn	mg	0.20	0.24
Copper, Cu	mg	0.017	0.045
Manganese, Mn	mg	0.155	0.143
Fluoride, F	mcg	47.5	3.2
Selenium, Se	mcg	0.7	0.1
Vitamins			
Vitamin C, total ascorbic acid	mg	3.6	5.9
Thiamin	mg	0.066	0.066
Riboflavin	mg	0.044	0.058
Niacin	mg	0.645	0.983
Pantothenic acid	mg	0.232	0.273
Vitamin B-6	mg	0.153	0.138
Folate, total	mcg	14	19
Folate, food	mcg	14	19
Folate, DFE	mcg_DFE	14	19

---

[80] Robertson J, Brydon WG, Tadesse K, Wenham P, Walls A, Eastwood MA. The effect of raw carrot on serum lipids and colon function. Am J Clin Nutr. 1979 Sep;32(9):1889-92.

Choline, total	mg	8.8	8.8
Betaine	mg	0.1	0.4
Vitamin A, RAE	mcg_RAE	852	835
Carotene, beta	mcg	8332	8285
Carotene, alpha	mcg	3776	3477
Vitamin A, IU	IU	17033	16706
Lycopene	mcg	0	1
Lutein + zeaxanthin	mcg	687	256
Vitamin E (alpha-tocopherol)	mg	1.03	0.66
Tocopherol, beta	mg	0.02	0.01
Vitamin K (phylloquinone)	mcg	13.7	13.2
Amino acids			
Tryptophan	g	0.010	0.012
Threonine	g	0.157	0.191
Isoleucine	g	0.063	0.077
Leucine	g	0.084	0.102
Lysine	g	0.083	0.101
Methionine	g	0.017	0.020
Cystine	g	0.068	0.083
Phenylalanine	g	0.050	0.061
Tyrosine	g	0.035	0.043
Valine	g	0.056	0.069
Arginine	g	0.075	0.091
Histidine	g	0.033	0.040
Alanine	g	0.093	0.113
Aspartic acid	g	0.156	0.190
Glutamic acid	g	0.301	0.366
Glycine	g	0.038	0.047
Proline	g	0.044	0.054
Serine	g	0.044	0.054

Bamboo Shoots (Zhú Sǔn Jiān, Sǔn Jiān)

Bamboo shoots are cooling and enter the Lung and Large Intestine channels. Bamboo shoots treat constipation and also heat type Lung and coughing disorders.

Bamboo shoots are contraindicated for patients with skin conditions and tumors. According to Chinese medicine theory, bamboo shoots grow rapidly and this functional characteristic may stimulate skin disorders and tumor growth.

Fresh bamboo shoots are available in Asian markets. Bamboo shoots are also sold in canned and dried forms. They are added to soups, boiled, pickled, fermented and stir-fried. Bamboo shoots are very low in fat, protein, carbohydrates, calories, contain no cholesterol and have an abundance of fiber. The high fiber content contributes to bamboo shoots' effectiveness in the treatment of constipation. Bamboo shoots lower cholesterol and are an appropriate food for the treatment of obesity due to the low carbohydrate and caloric content.[81]

Papaya

Papaya is sweet, neutral, and enters the Stomach and Large Intestine channels. Two major varieties have either red-orange or yellow flesh when ripe. Both varieties are picked green. Green papaya is tender, firm and is commonly prepared in salads and sautés. Papayas contain papain, an enzyme helpful in the digestion of proteins that has anti-inflammatory properties. Papayas are rich in vitamin C, folate, potassium, fiber, vitamin A, vitamin E and vitamin K. Orange-red papaya is rich in carotene, an antioxidant.

- Recipe for children with a chronic cough: Chuan Bei Dun Mu Gua. Dun is translated as double-boiling. Cut in half a ripe or half-ripened papaya and remove the seeds. Fill one of the halves with Mu Gua and crushed Chuan Bei Mu. The Mu Gua liquefies when double boiled. Double-boil the papaya half while covered with a lid. The Mu Gua adds flavor and has a moistening property to promote Jin Ye fluids. Mu Gua also has enzymes that assist with the digestion of proteins. Mu Gua has significant nutritional value and has antioxidant properties.

- Recipe to promote lactation or to treat weakness of the feet: Mu Gua Hua Shen Ju Pi Tang. Combine and cook raw peanuts (including the skin), Mu Gua, pork feet, and papaya. In Chinese medicine theory, the white juice of the ripe papaya is connected with the function of lactation. In general, rich gelatinous foods tend to promote lactation. The

---

[81] Eun-Jin Park, Ph.D., Deok-Young Jhon, Ph.D.. Effects of bamboo shoot consumption on lipid profiles and bowel function in healthy young women. Volume 25, Issue 7, Pages 723-728 (July 2009).

pork feet add to the strengthening of the feet function according to the Chinese medicine theory of 'foot to foot'.

- Help the skin remain smooth and beautiful with fresh ripe papaya juice. This is a popular offering with street venders in Taiwan.

Loofah (Si Gua)

Loofah is a green vegetable that is similar in appearance to cucumber. Loofah is also used as a sponge when allowed to mature and after processing removes all contents except for the fibers. The fiber-only preparation is sweet, neutral and is used in herbal medicine preparations for topical and internal applications.

As a green vegetable, loofah is tender and green when young. As it ages, loofah becomes tough, rough and brown. The green loofah is sweet, cooling, enters the Lung, Liver, and Stomach channels; and can be consumed regularly. Si Gua refers to the green vegetable and Si Gua Luo refers to the fiber-only preparation. Si Gua and Si Gua Lou have similar functions although Si Gua Lou has a stronger medicinal function because it has aged.

According to Chinese medicine theory, the network of visible fibers in loofah indicate that Si Gua and Si Gua Lou open the channels, peripheral channels and collaterals. This property is helpful in the treatment of bi zheng (painful obstruction syndrome) and pain due to phlegm, qi or blood stagnation. Si Gua and Si Gua Lou invigorate the blood and are helpful in the treatment of injuries. They dissolve phlegm and treat coughing with copious amounts of phlegm and also pain due to injuries incurred from a chronic cough. Si Gua and Si Gua Lou promote lactation and also clear heat toxins in the treatment of breast abscesses.

Learn more in the second volume. *Volume 2* **features more individual food items and special recipes for specific ailments.**

Special Recipes and Food Treatments in Chinese Medicine Dietetics, Volume 2

Headache Recipes
- Wind-Cold Headache
- Wind-Heat Headache
- Damp Headache
- Phlegm Dampness Headache
- Liver Yang Uprising Headache
- Qi Deficiency or Yin Deficiency Headache
- Headache due to Trauma
- Food Stagnation Headache

Respiratory System Recipes
- Common Cold Recipes
- Bronchitis Recipes

Digestive System Recipes
- Cold and Deficient Stomach Pain
- Cold Stomach Disorders
- Bleeding Stomach Ulcer, Gastroenteritis, Ulcerative Colitis, or Nonspecific Bleeding in the GI System
- Chronic Loose Stool, Diarrhea, Chronic Dysentery, Colitis, or IBS (Irritable Bowel Syndrome) with Underlying Spleen Qi Deficiency
- Constipation

Urinary System Recipes

Diabetes Recipes

Overweight and Obesity Recipes

Skin Disorder Recipes

High Blood Pressure Recipes

Additional Foods In
Chinese Medicine Dietetics, Volume 2

Fruits, Vegetables, Herbs

Apple	Grapes	Orange
Asian Pear	Honey Dew Melon	Peach
Asparagus	Jin Zhen Cai (Daylily	Persimmon
Avocado	Flower)	Pi Pa (Loquat)
Banana	Kiwi	Pineapple
Beet	Kumquat	Pomelo
Broccoli	Lemon	Prunes and Plums
Cabbage	Lime	Shi Liu (Pomegranate)
Chard	Mango	Spinach
Cherry	Mulberry	Tangerine
Fig	Onion	Tomatoes

Nuts

Chestnut	Pine Nut	Sweet Almond (Xing Ren)
Ginkgo	Pumpkin Seeds	Walnuts
Peanut	Sesame Seed	Young Coconut

Seafood

Abalone	Jellyfish	Seaweed
Carp Fish	Oyster	Shark Fin
Catfish	Sea Cucumber	Shrimp
Frog	Sea Snake	Turtle

Bird Meat and Products

Bird's Nest	Eggs	Pigeon
Black Bone Chicken	Goose	Quail
Duck	Ostrich	Turkey

Meats and Dairy

Beef	Milk	Rabbit
Venison	Pork	Snake
Goat		

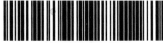

Made in the USA
Lexington, KY
03 February 2012